FIRST EDITION

ISBN: 978-1-716-56750-6

I0499931

Introduction

Translation Medic was created in 2020 by career EMS professionals for EMS professionals. The authors found that there was a need for a translation aid that was easy to use, and catered towards EMS. The authors hope that Translation Medic can be utilized to streamline and improve care of minority communities. The authors of Translation Medic are striving to improve the product to fit the needs of modern EMS providers. If you have any suggestions and/or comments please email them to: Translationmedic@gmail.com.

Cantonese/Mandarin Translation

Alert & Oriented Questions 2
Chief Complaints 3
Chest Pain 4-5
Abdominal Pain 6-7
Other Pains 8-9
Breathing Difficulty 10-11
Nausea & Vomiting 12-13
Syncope 14-15
ALOC/Stroke 16-17
Dizziness/Headache 18-19
Fall 20
Traumatic injury other than fall 21-22
Miscellaneous Questions 23
Pertinent Medical History List 24
Medications List 25
Allergies List 26
Intervention Phrases 27

Spanish Translation

Alert & Oriented Questions 29
Chief Complaints 30
Chest Pain 31-32
Abdominal Pain 33-34
Other Pains 35-36
Breathing Difficulty 37-38
Nausea & Vomiting 39-40
Syncope 41-42
ALOC/Stroke 43-44
Dizziness/Headache 45-46
Fall 47
Traumatic injury other than fall 48-49
Miscellaneous Questions 50
Pertinent Medical History List 51
Medications List 52
Allergies List 53
Intervention Phrases 54

Russian Translation

Cantonese/Mandarin

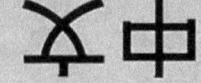
中文

Hello I am a medical professional. I do not speak your language, but I will be using this translation guide to help me. Please read the question and point to the correct choice

你好。我是一位專業急求救員.。我將會用這本中英文翻譯指南與你交流。請回覆這些問題(請指出答案)

Alert & Oriented Questions

What is your name?		名字？	
Where are we now? **請指出你現在哪裡？**	House 家裡	Restaurant 餐廳	Outside 戶外
	Store 商店	Ambulance 救護車裡	Other 其它地方

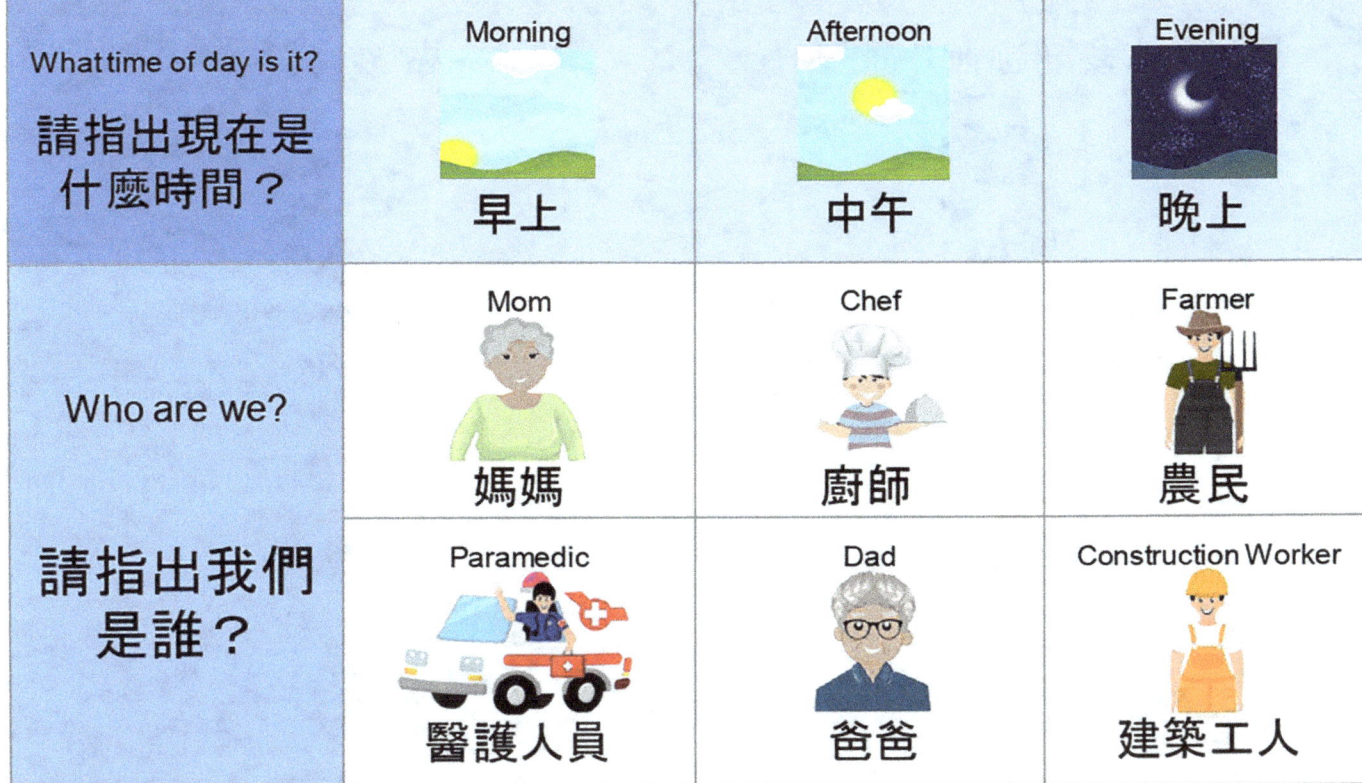

What time of day is it? 請指出現在是什麼時間？	Morning 早上	Afternoon 中午	Evening 晚上
Who are we? 請指出我們是誰？	Mom 媽媽	Chef 廚師	Farmer 農民
	Paramedic 醫護人員	Dad 爸爸	Construction Worker 建築工人

2

Chief Complaints

What's going on today?	請指出哪裡不舒服？
Chest Pain | p. 4-5 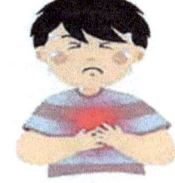 心痛	Abdominal Pain | p. 6-7 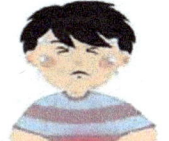 腹痛(肚子痛)
Other Pains | p.8-9 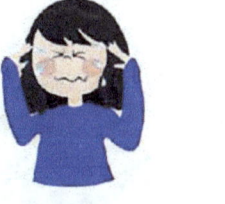 其他疼痛	Breathing Problem | p.10-11 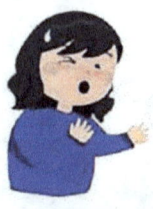 呼吸問題

Nausea/Vomiting | p. 12-13	Syncope | p.14-15	ALOC/Stroke | p.16-17
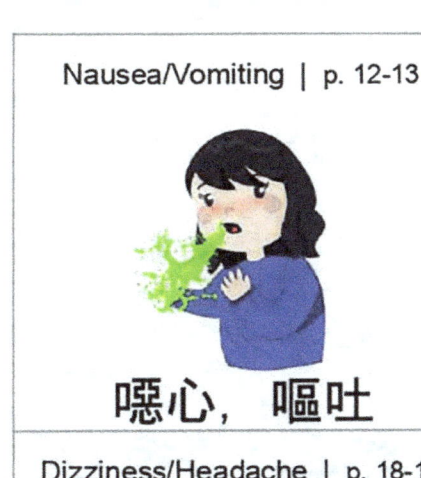 噁心，嘔吐	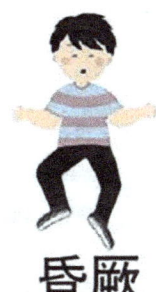 昏厥	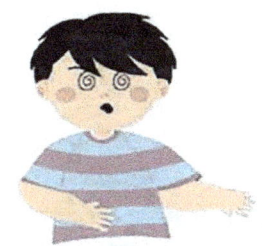 表現不正常，中風
Dizziness/Headache | p. 18-19	Fall | p. 20	Traumatic injury | p. 21-22
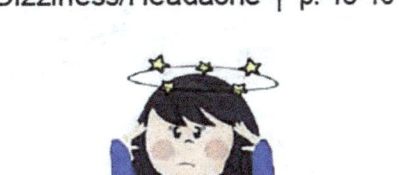 頭暈，頭痛	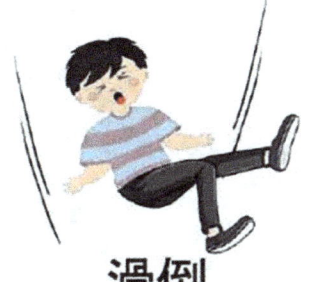 滑倒	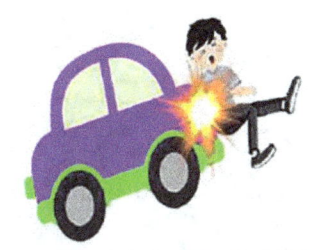 摔倒以外的創傷

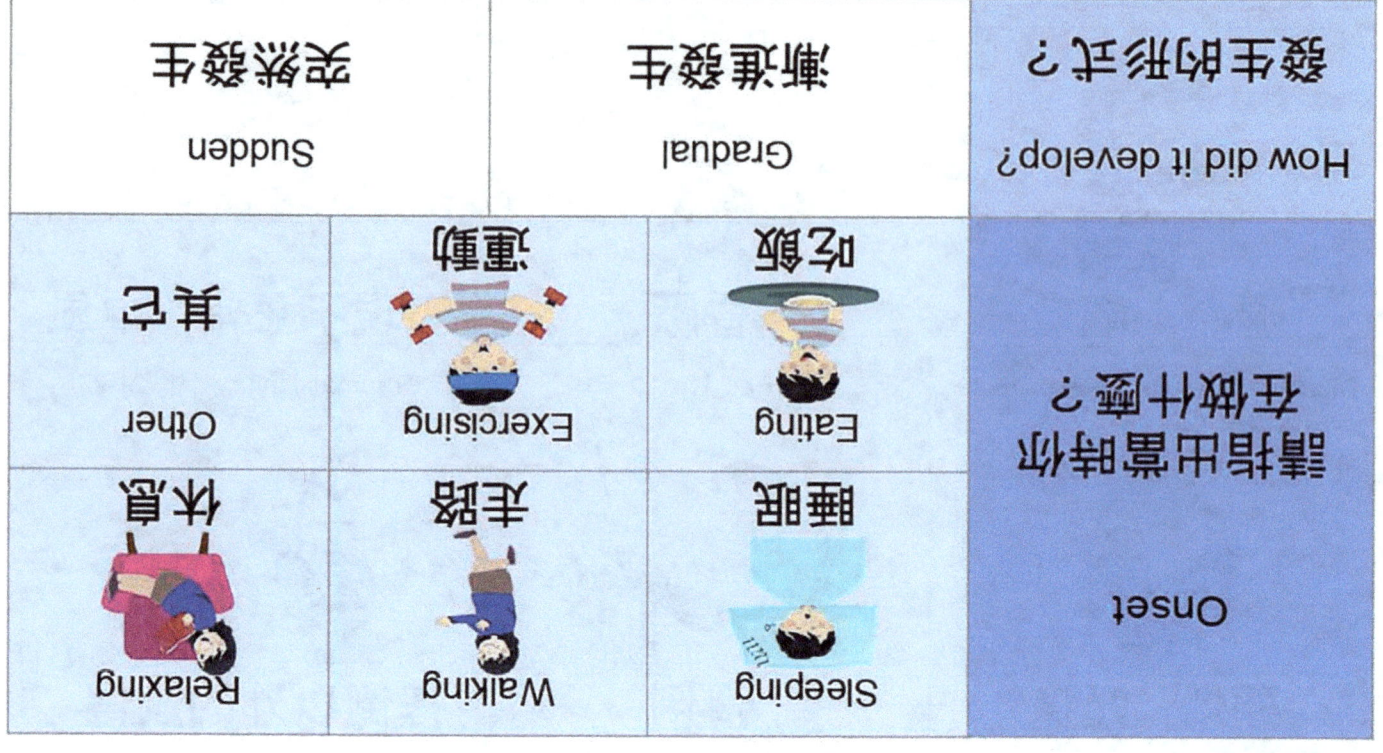

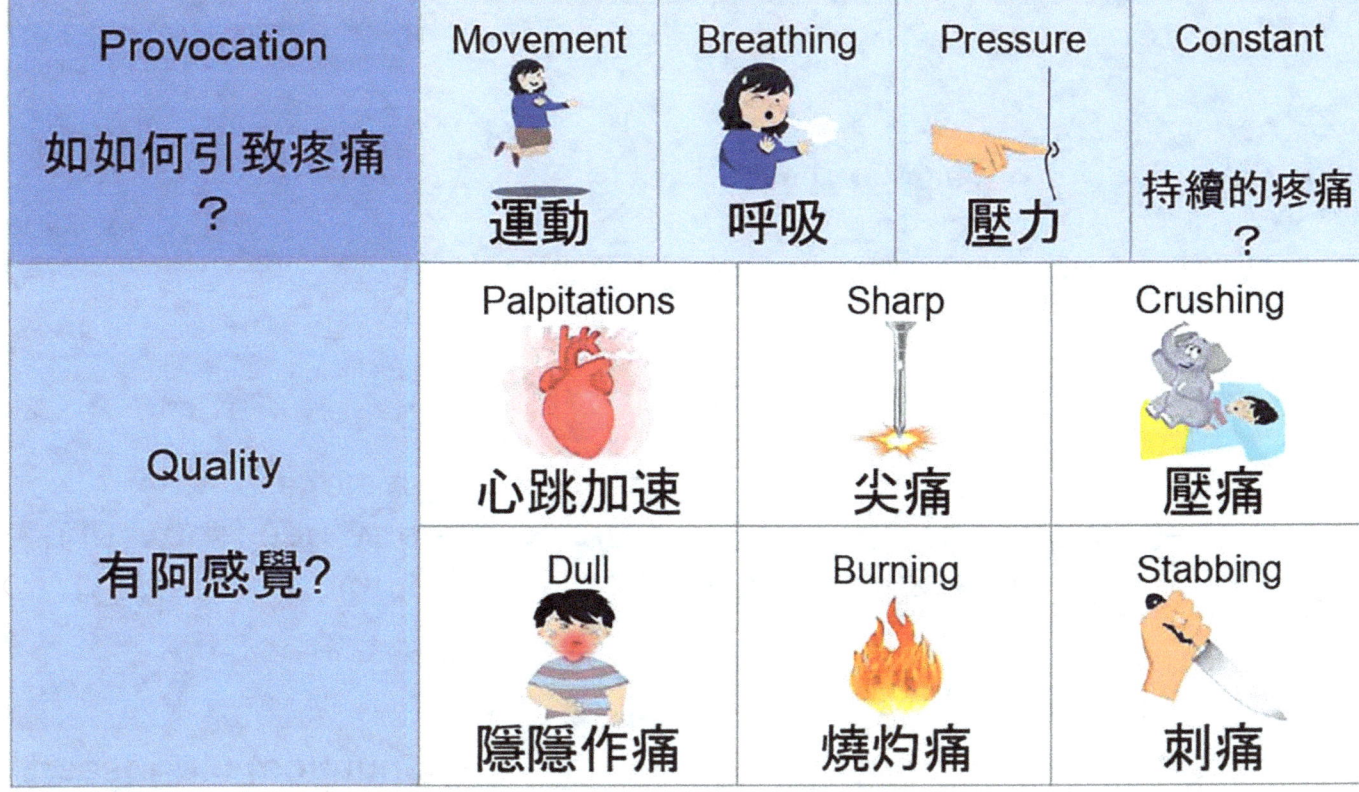

Chest Pain (continued)

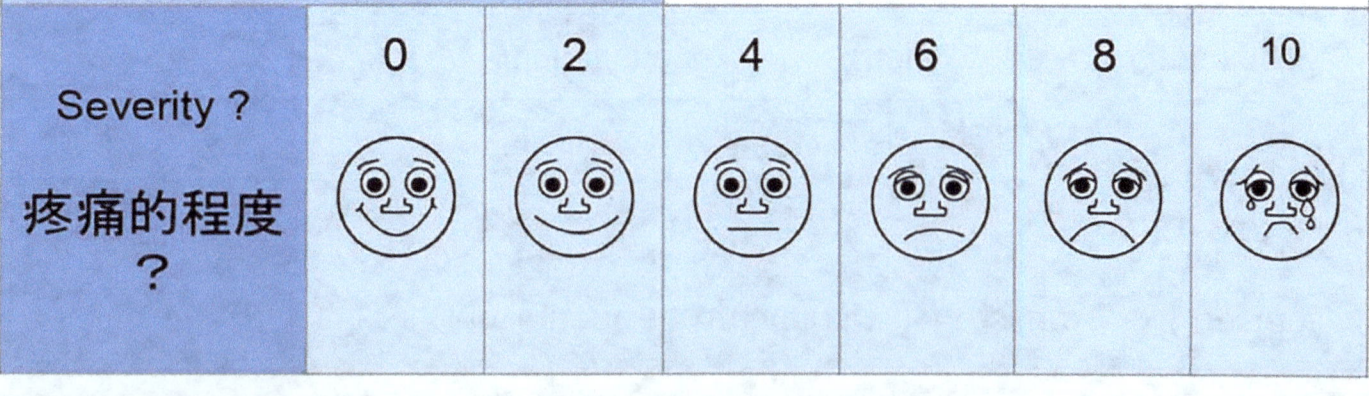

Radiation/ Point to where it hurts most and where the pain travels to	請指出最痛的部位，疼痛放射到的地方				
Severity ? 疼痛的程度 ？	0	2	4	6	8	10

Time 疼痛時間多久？	10 Mins 10分鐘	Half Hour 半小時	1 Hour 1小時
	2 Hours 2小時	3 Hours 3 小時	>4 Hours 4小時以上

Pertinent Negatives/ Are you having any of the following 你有以下症狀嗎？	No X 沒有	Abdominal Pain 腹痛	Breathing Difficulty 呼吸困難
		Nausea/Vomiting 噁心、嘔吐	Other Pains 其它

5

Abdominal Pain

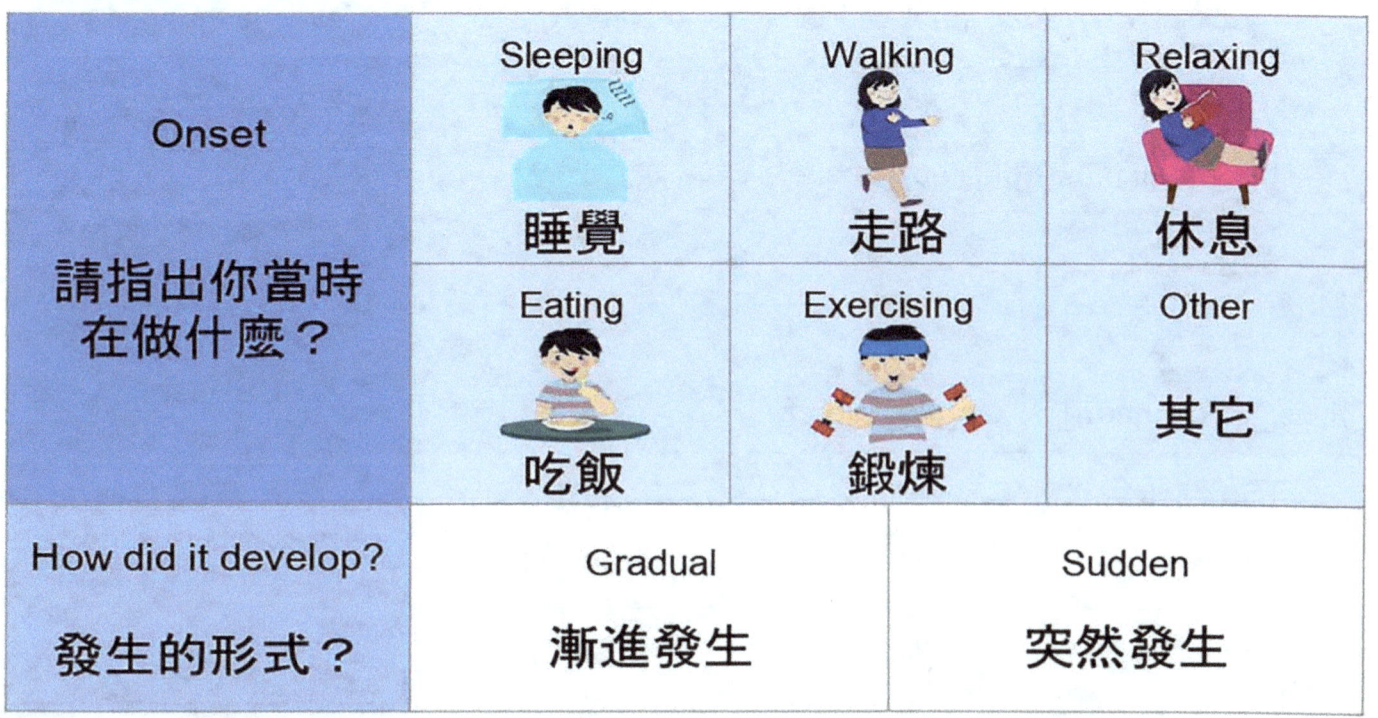

Onset 請指出你當時 在做什麼？	Sleeping 睡覺	Walking 走路	Relaxing 休息
	Eating 吃飯	Exercising 鍛煉	Other 其它
How did it develop? 發生的形式？	Gradual 漸進發生		Sudden 突然發生

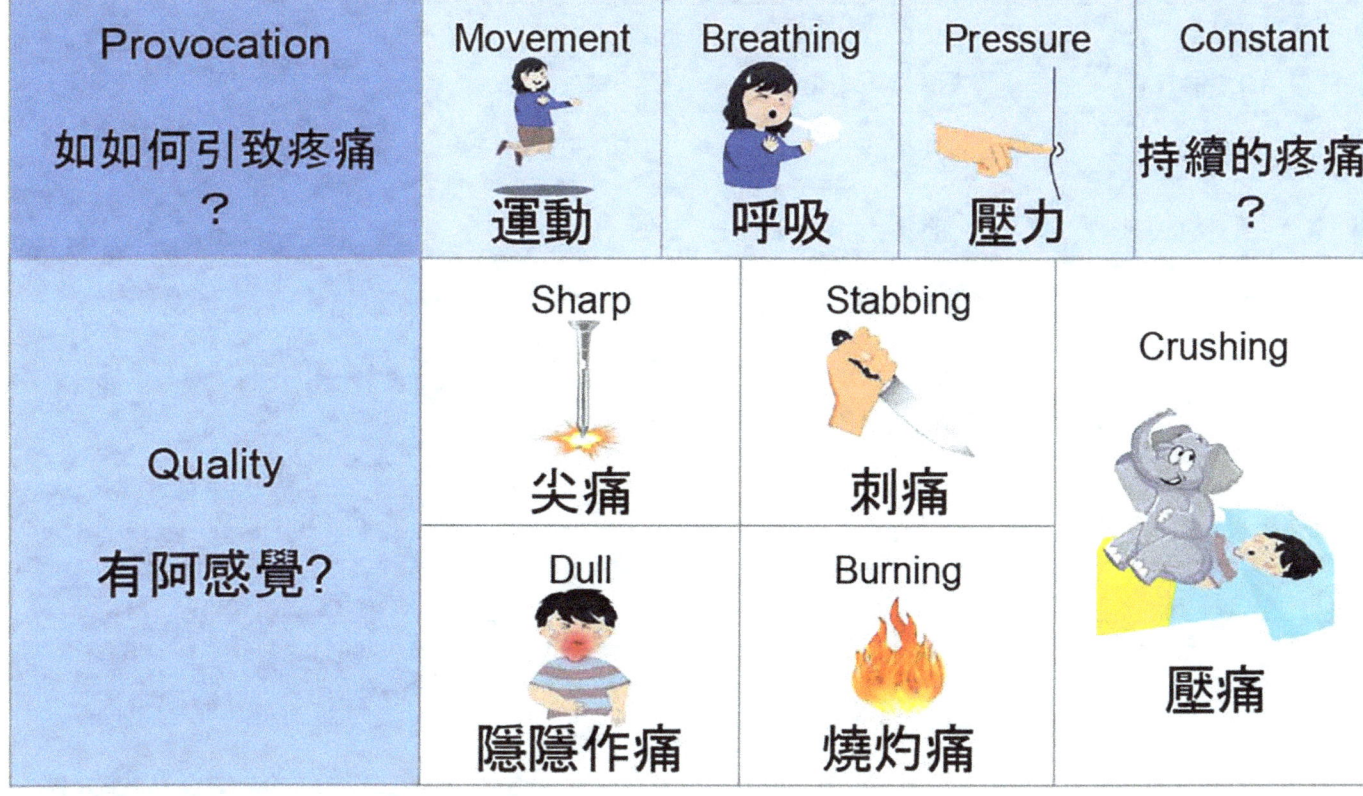

Provocation 如如何引致疼痛？	Movement 運動	Breathing 呼吸	Pressure 壓力	Constant 持續的疼痛？
Quality 有阿感覺？	Sharp 尖痛 / Dull 隱隱作痛	Stabbing 刺痛 / Burning 燒灼痛		Crushing 壓痛

6

Abdominal Pain (continued)

Radiation/ Point to where it hurts most and where the pain travels to	請指出最痛的部位，疼痛放射到的地方					
Severity ? 疼痛的程度 ？	0 ☺	2 ☺	4 😐	6 ☹	8 ☹	10 😢
Time 疼痛時間多久 ？	10 Mins 10分鐘		Half Hour 半小時		1 Hour 1小時	
	2 Hours 2小時		3 Hours 3 小時		>4 Hours 4小時以上	

Is there any chance you are pregnant? 有懷孕嗎？	Yes ｜ 是 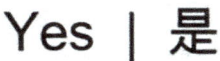	No ｜ 沒有 X
Pertinent Negatives/ Are you having any of the following/你有以下症狀嗎？	**No** X 沒有 / **Abdominal Pain**  腹痛 / **Nausea/Vomiting** 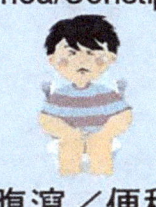 噁心、嘔吐 / **Diarrhea/Constipation** 腹瀉／便秘	**Breathing Difficulty** 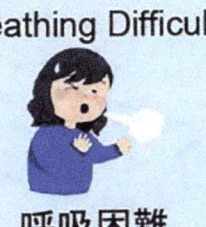 呼吸困難 / **Other Pains** 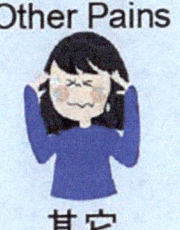 其它

7

Other Pains

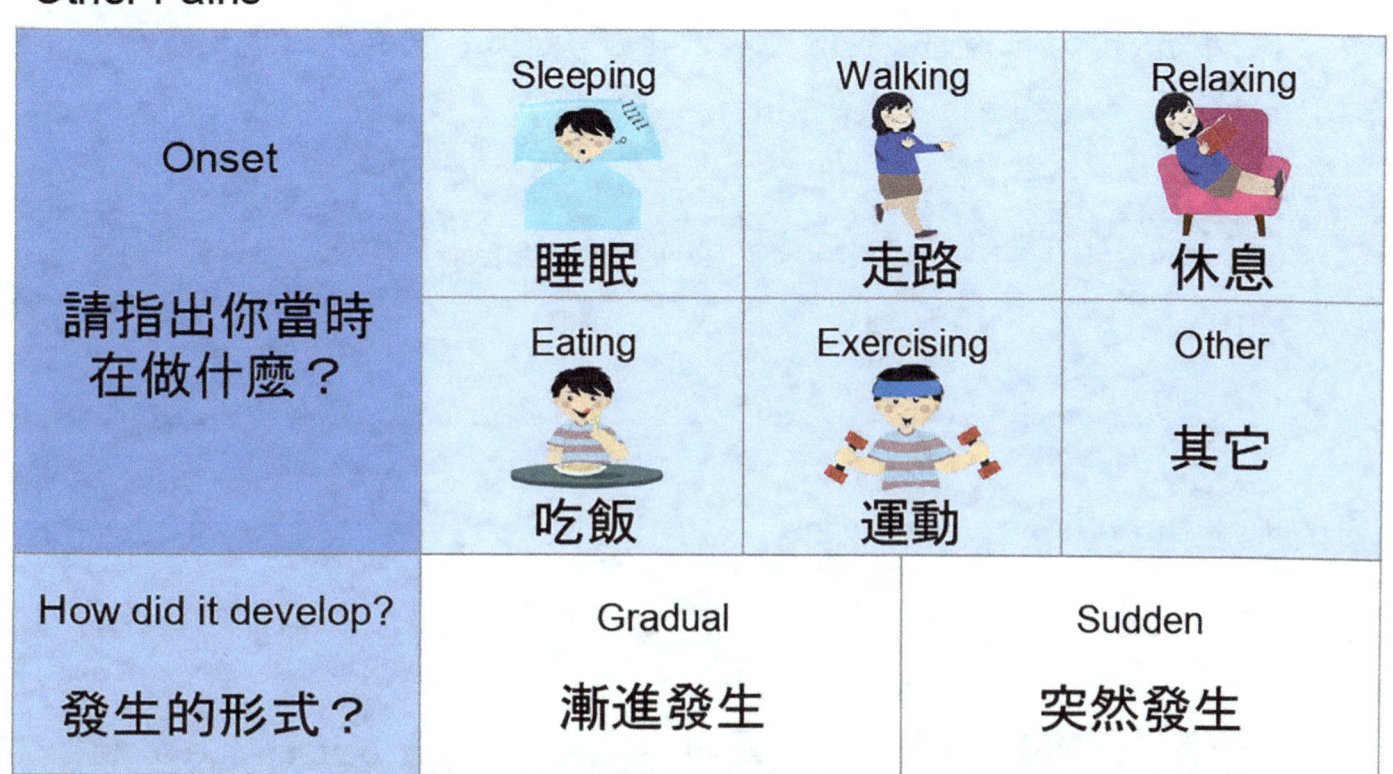

Onset 請指出你當時在做什麼？	Sleeping 睡眠	Walking 走路	Relaxing 休息
	Eating 吃飯	Exercising 運動	Other 其它
How did it develop? 發生的形式？	Gradual 漸進發生		Sudden 突然發生

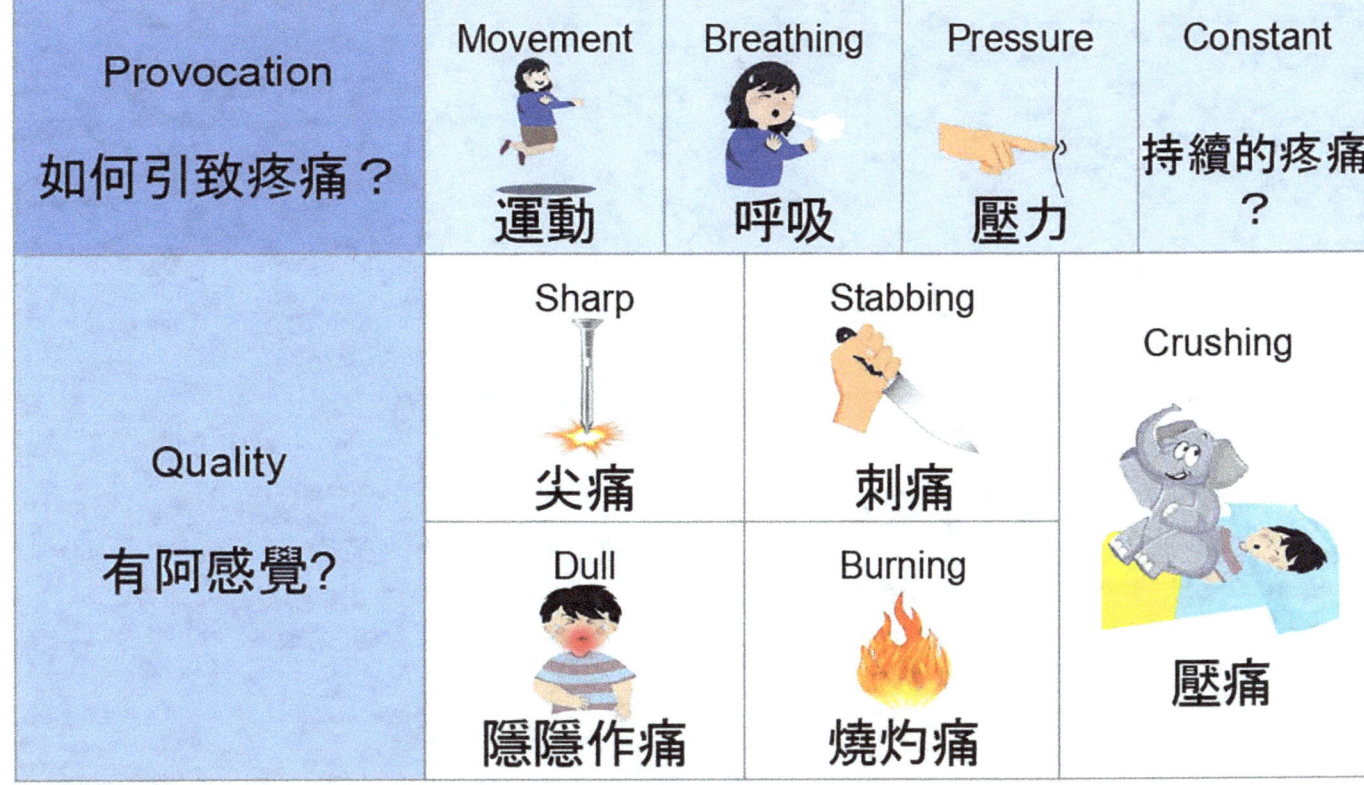

Provocation 如何引致疼痛？	Movement 運動	Breathing 呼吸	Pressure 壓力	Constant 持續的疼痛？
Quality 有阿感覺？	Sharp 尖痛 / Dull 隱隱作痛	Stabbing 刺痛 / Burning 燒灼痛		Crushing 壓痛

Other Pains (continued)

Radiation: Point to where it hurts most and where the pain travels to	請指出最痛的部位，疼痛放射到的地方？

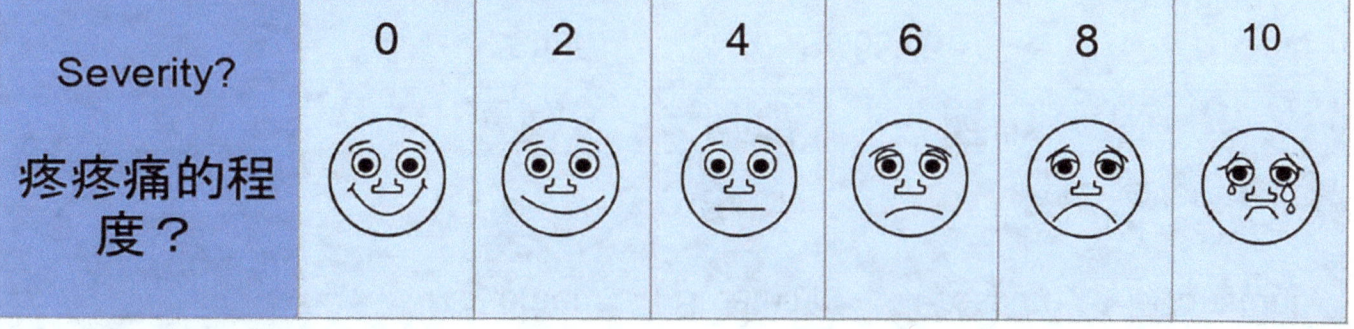

Severity? 疼疼痛的程度？	0	2	4	6	8	10

Time 疼痛時間多久？	10 Mins 10分鐘	Half Hour 半小時	1 Hour 1小時
	2 Hours 2小時	3 Hours 3 小時	>4 Hours 4小時以上
Pertinent Negatives/ Are you having any of the following 你有以下症狀嗎？	No X 沒有	Abdominal Pain 腹痛	Breathing Difficulty 呼吸困難
	Nausea/Vomiting 噁心，嘔吐	Chest Pain 心痛	Syncope 昏厥

Shortness of Breath

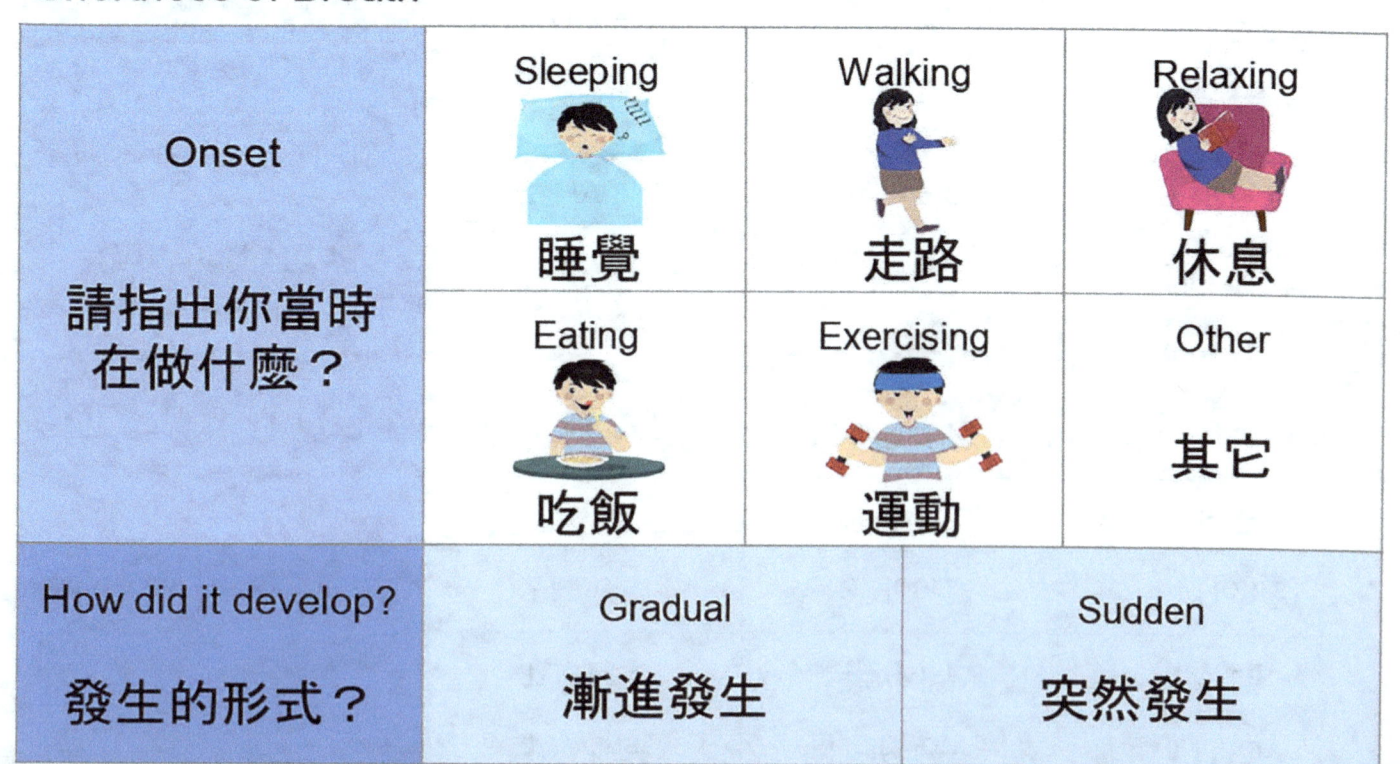

Onset 請指出你當時 在做什麼？	Sleeping 睡覺	Walking 走路	Relaxing 休息
	Eating 吃飯	Exercising 運動	Other 其它

How did it develop? 發生的形式？	Gradual 漸進發生	Sudden 突然發生

Do you have associated chest pain? 胸痛？心痛？	Yes ｜ 有 ✔	No ｜ 沒有 ✗	
Sputum: Are you coughing, what color is your phlegm? 你有沒有咳嗽？痰是什麼顏色？	None ✗ 沒有	Dry Cough 乾咳	White 白色
	Yellow 黃色	Green 綠色	Pink/Bloody 粉紅色／血紅色

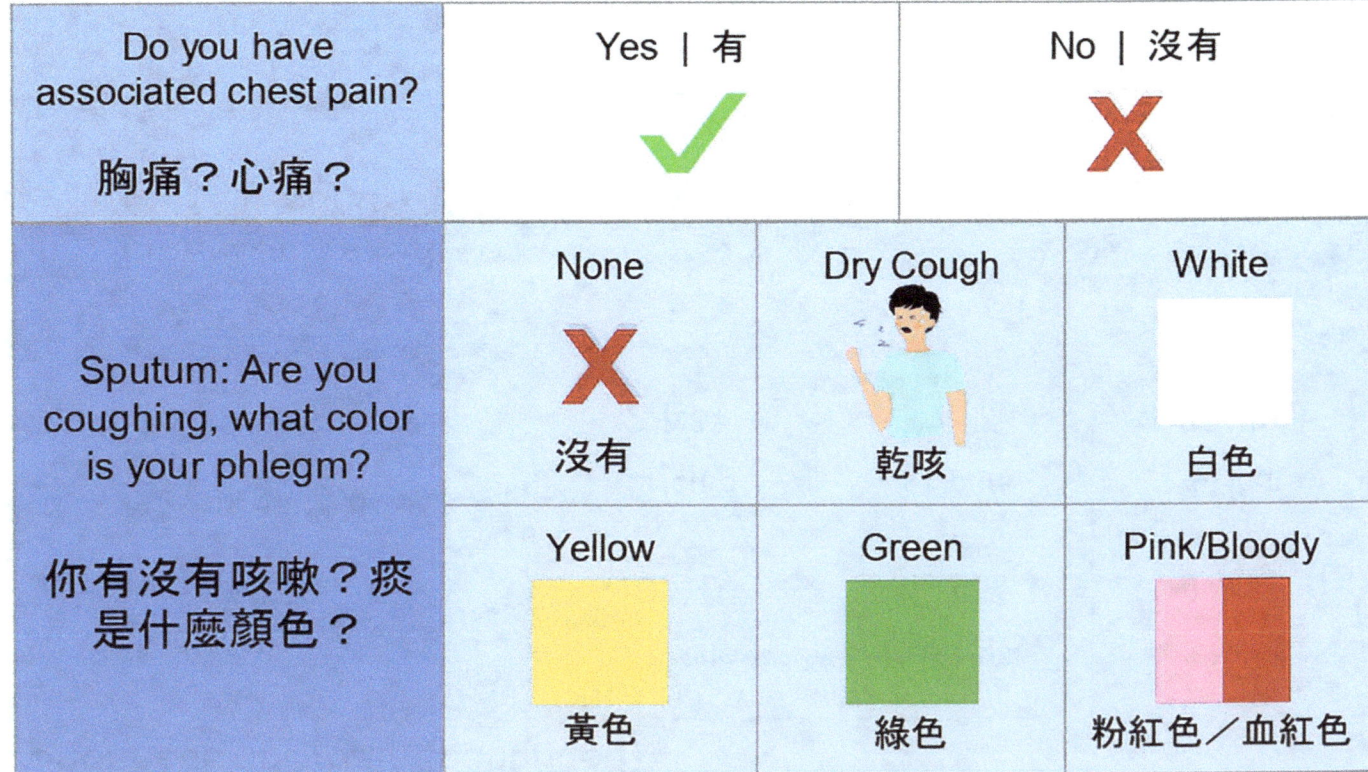

10

Shortness of Breath (continued)

Time 疼痛時間多久？	10 Mins 10分鐘	Half Hour 半小時	1 Hour 1小時
	2 Hours 2小時	3 Hours 3 小時	>4 Hours 4小時以上

Exertion: Does movement and exercise make it worse? 如果運動病情會惡化嗎？	Yes ｜ 會 ✔	No ｜ 不會 ✗

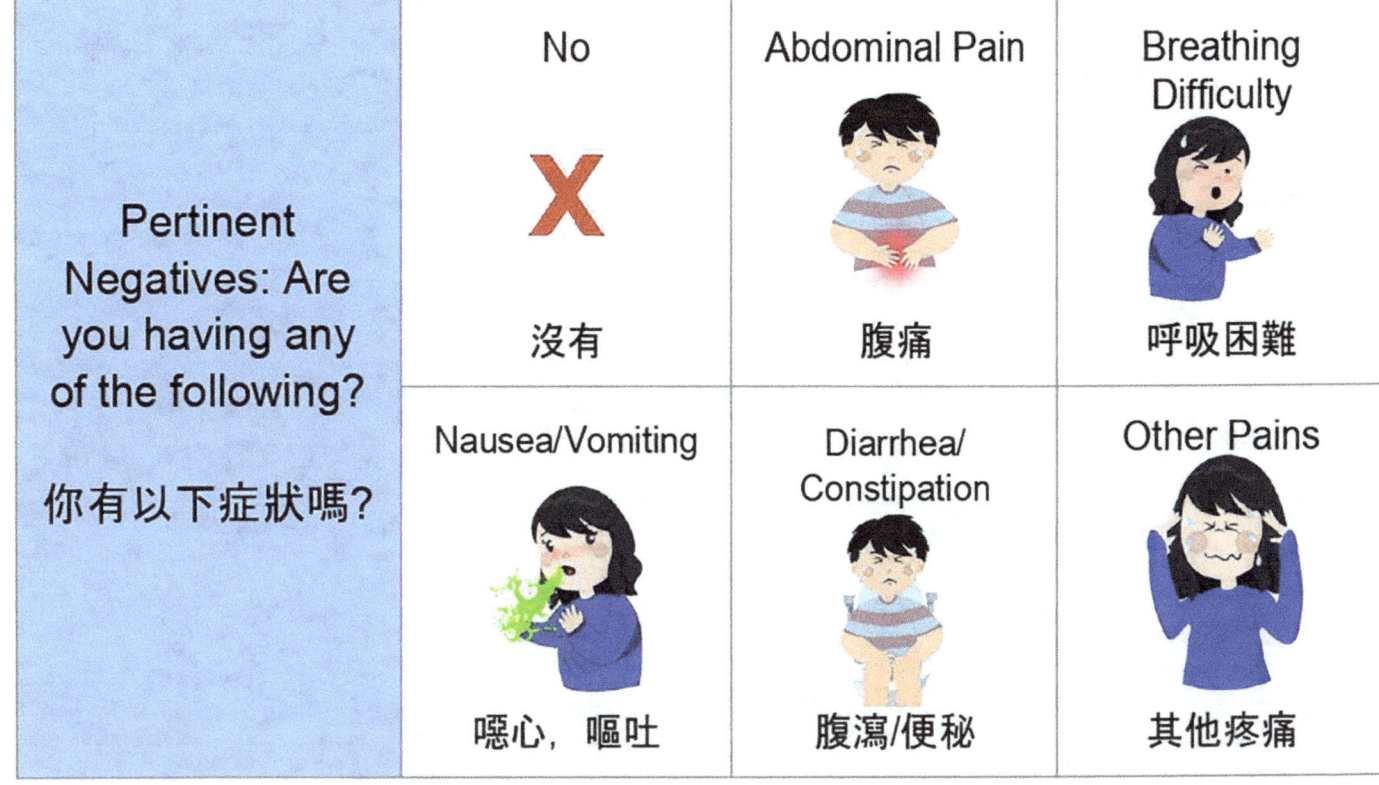

Pertinent Negatives: Are you having any of the following?

你有以下症狀嗎?

No	Abdominal Pain	Breathing Difficulty
X		
沒有	腹痛	呼吸困難
Nausea/Vomiting	Diarrhea/ Constipation	Other Pains
噁心, 嘔吐	腹瀉/便秘	其他疼痛

Nausea and Vomiting

Onset 請指出你當時在做什麼？	Sleeping 睡眠	Walking 走路	Relaxing 休息
	Eating 吃飯	Exercising 運動	Other 其它
Is there any blood in your vomit? 嘔吐物有血嗎？	Yes | 有 ✔		No | 沒有 ✗

Time 疼痛時間多久？	10 Mins 10分鐘	Half Hour 半小時	1 Hour 1小時
	2 Hours 2小時	3 Hours 3 小時	>4 Hours 4小時以上

Are you having abdominal pain? 你有肚子痛嗎？	Yes ｜ 有 ✔		No ｜ 沒有 ✗

Are you pregnant? 有懷孕嗎？	Yes ｜ 是 ✔ How many months? 懷孕多久？		No ｜ 沒有 ✗

12

Nausea and Vomiting (continued)

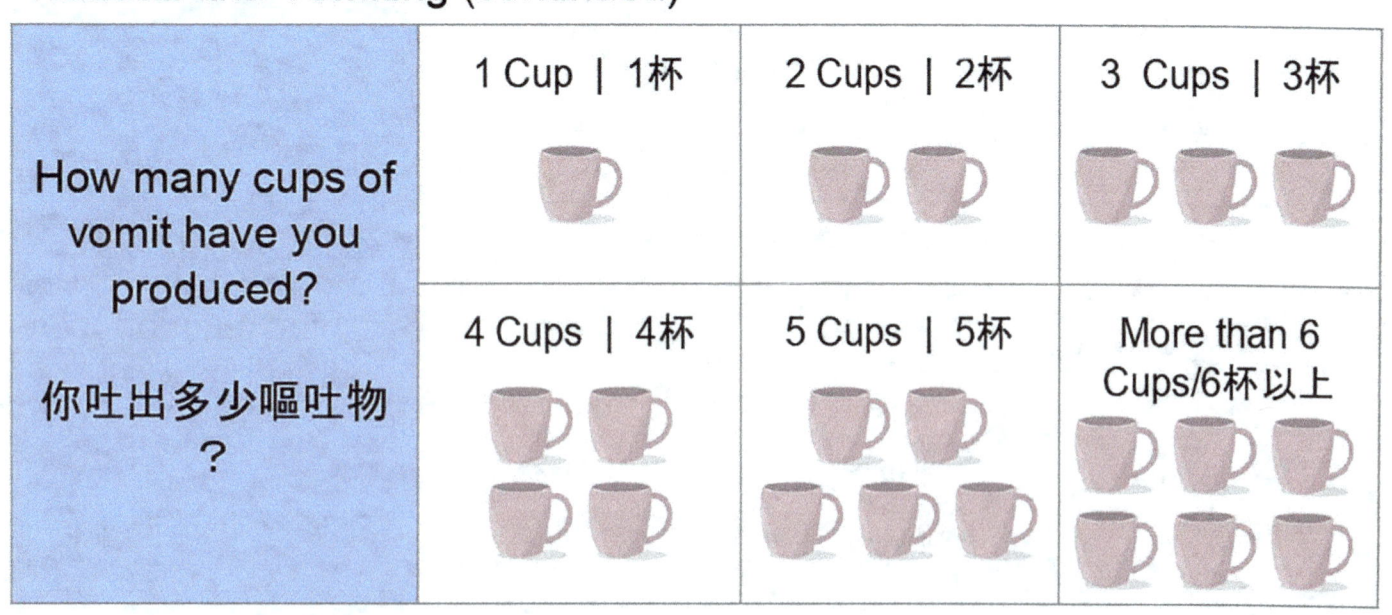

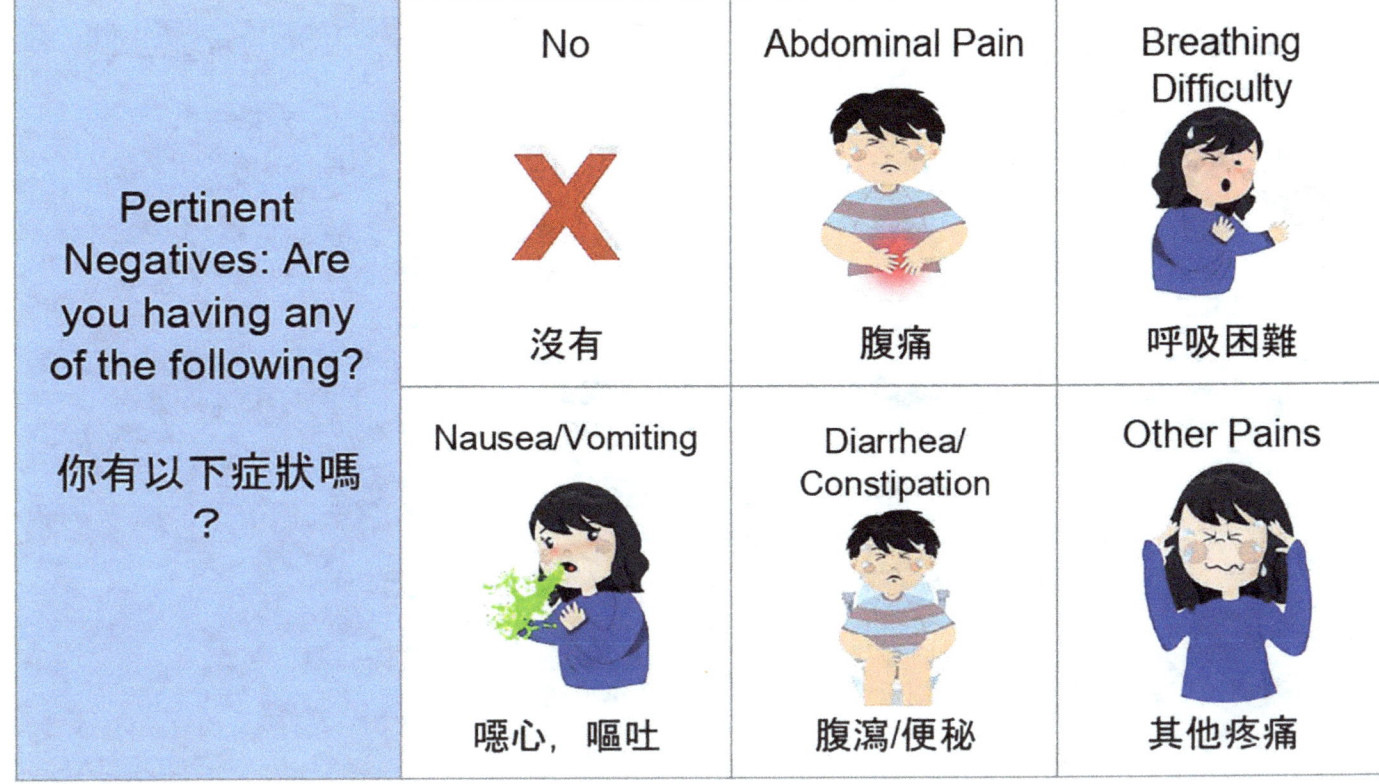

Pertinent Negatives: Are you having any of the following?

你有以下症狀嗎？

No	Abdominal Pain	Breathing Difficulty
X		
沒有	腹痛	呼吸困難
Nausea/Vomiting	Diarrhea/Constipation	Other Pains
噁心，嘔吐	腹瀉/便秘	其他疼痛

Syncope

Onset 請指出你當時在做什麼?	Sleeping 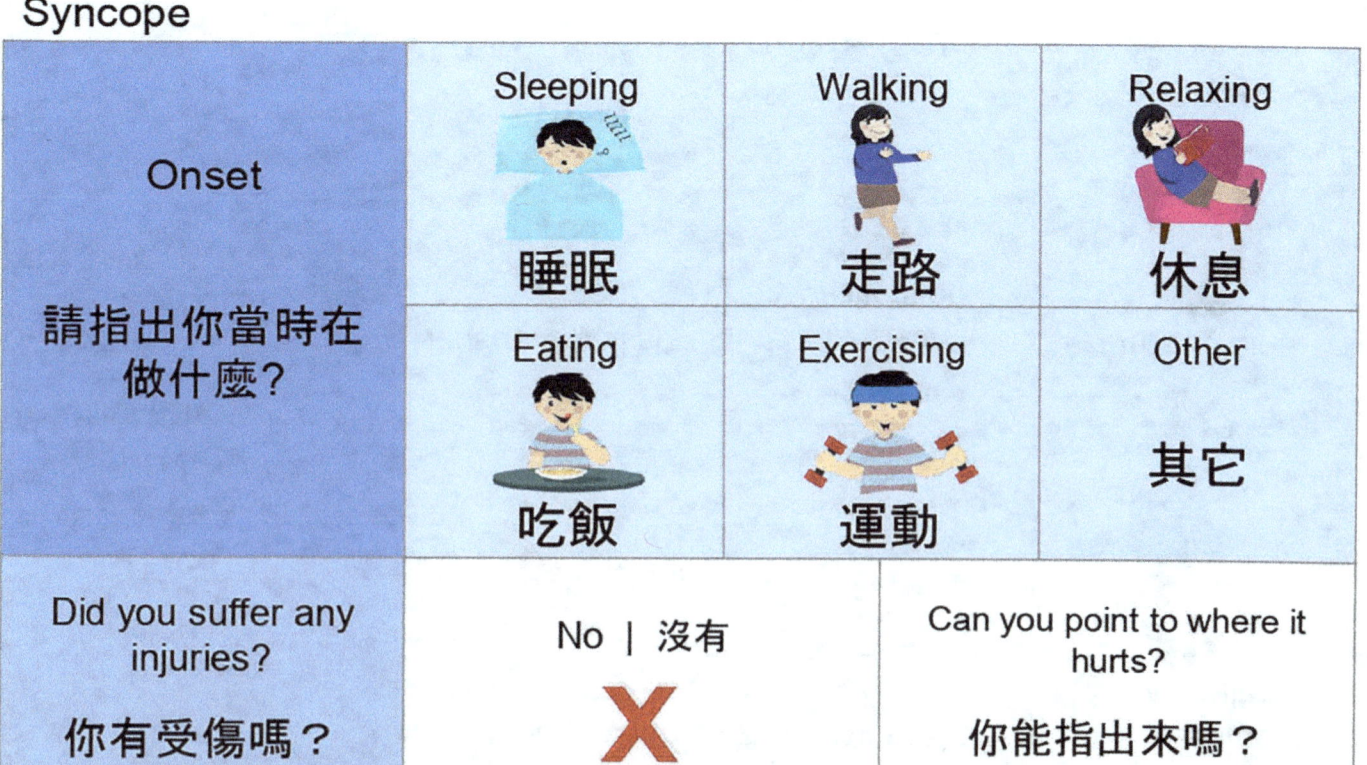睡眠	Walking 走路	Relaxing 休息
	Eating 吃飯	Exercising 運動	Other 其它
Did you suffer any injuries? 你有受傷嗎?	No ｜ 沒有 **X**		Can you point to where it hurts? 你能指出來嗎?

Time	10 Mins	Half Hour	1 Hour
疼痛時間多久？	10分鐘	半小時	1小時
	2 Hours	3 Hours	>4 Hours
	2小時	3 小時	4小時以上
What symptoms did you have prior? 事先感覺怎麼樣？	Felt Fine 沒有感覺	Chest Pain 心痛	Abdominal Pain 腹痛
	Shortness of Breath 呼吸困難	Nausea/Vomiting 噁心，嘔吐	Headache 頭痛

14

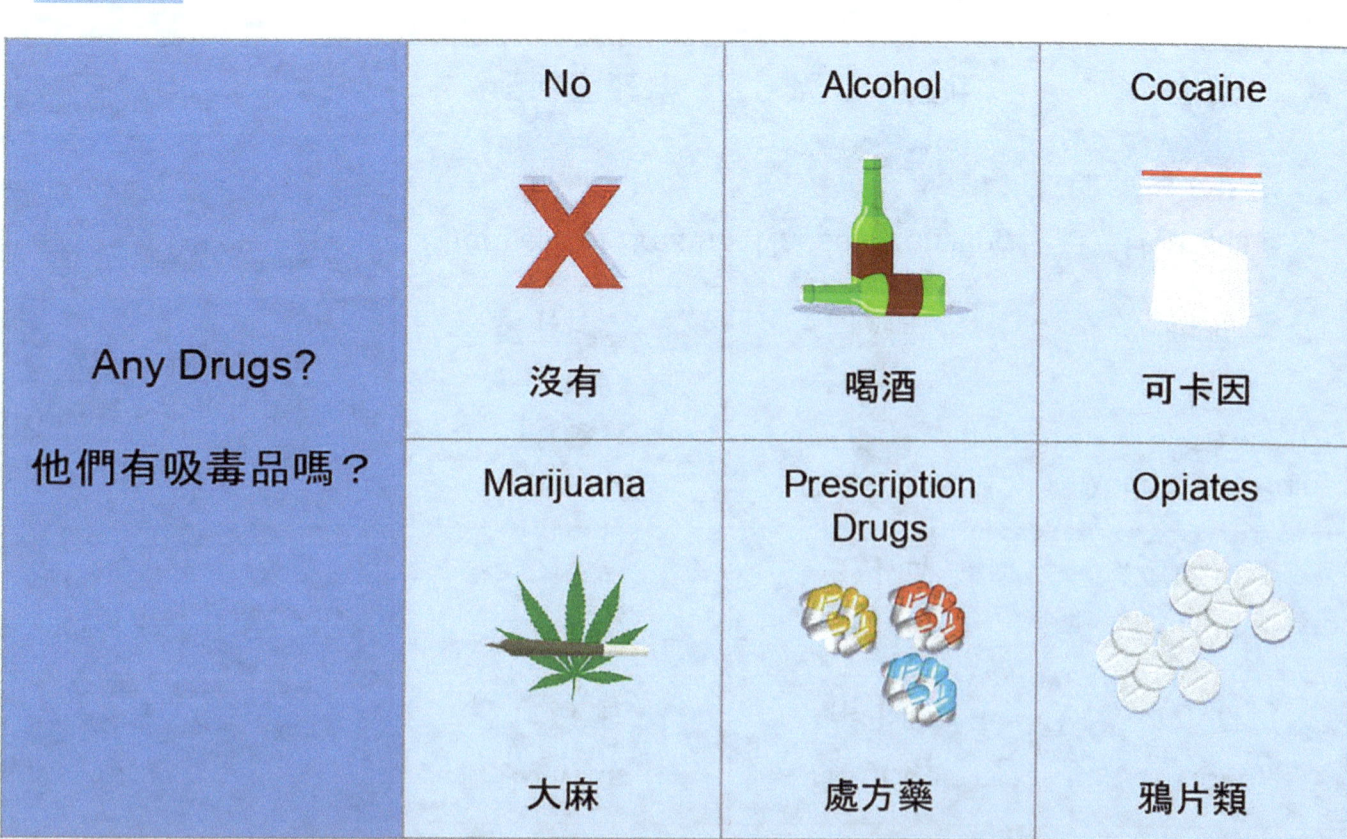

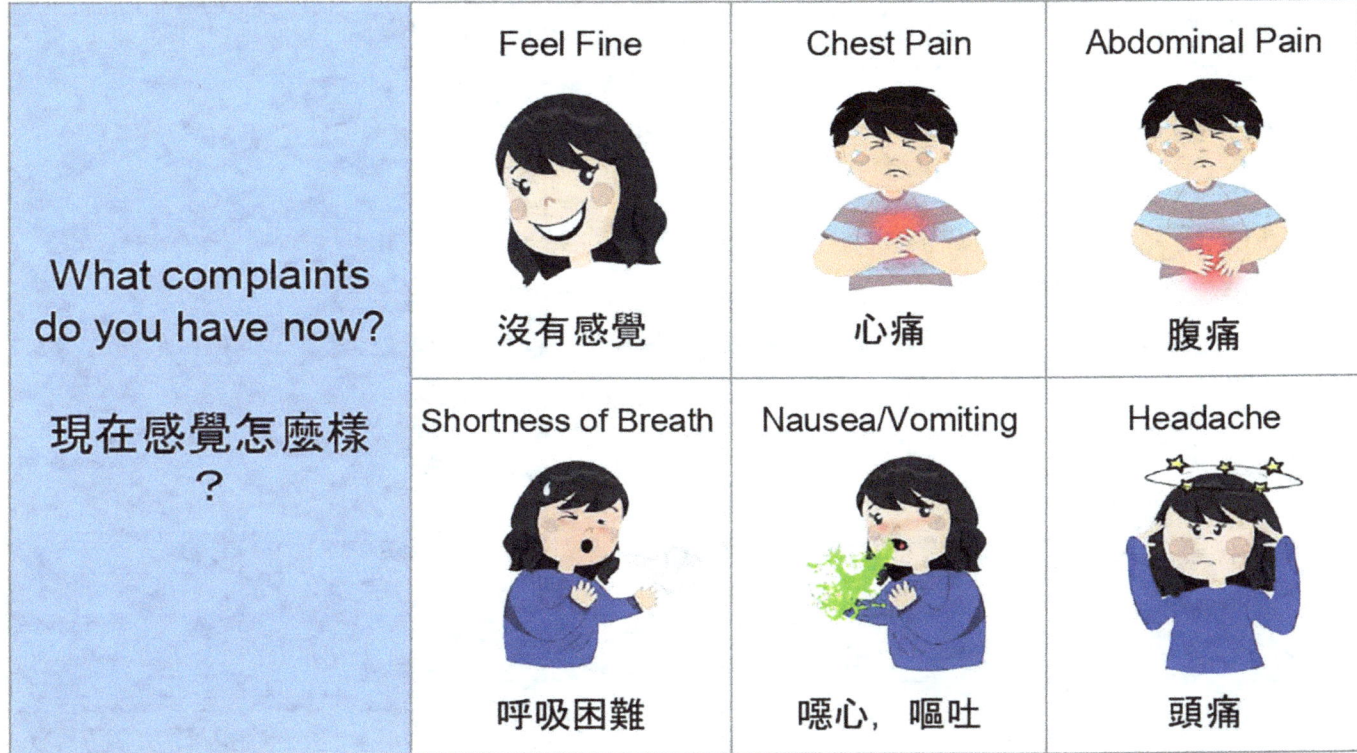

What complaints do you have now?

現在感覺怎麼樣？

Feel Fine	Chest Pain	Abdominal Pain
沒有感覺	心痛	腹痛
Shortness of Breath	Nausea/Vomiting	Headache
呼吸困難	噁心，嘔吐	頭痛

ALOC/Stroke

How is the patient normally?	通常他們情況如何？請指出	Yes/是 No/不是
Able to ambulate?	可以自己走動嗎？	Yes/是 No/不是
Know who they are?	知道自己是誰嗎？	Yes/是 No/不是
Know where they are?	知道自己在哪裡嗎？	Yes/是 No/不是
Know what year it is?	知道是哪一年嗎？	Yes/是 No/不是
Know what is going on?	知道發生什麼事情嗎？	Yes/是 No/不是
Did they hit their head?	有撞到頭嗎？請指出	Yes/是 No/不是

F	Can you smile for me?	你可以對我微笑嗎？		
A	Can you stick both arms out and close your eyes?	你能閉上眼睛伸出雙臂嗎？		
S	Can you say: I like to eat spaghetti?	你能說：我喜歡吃義大利面嗎？		
T	When were they last seen normal? 什麼時間是正常的？	10 Mins 10分鐘	Half Hour 半小時	1 Hour 1小時
		2-4 Hours 2-4小時	4-24 Hours 4-24 小時	>24 Hours 24小時以上

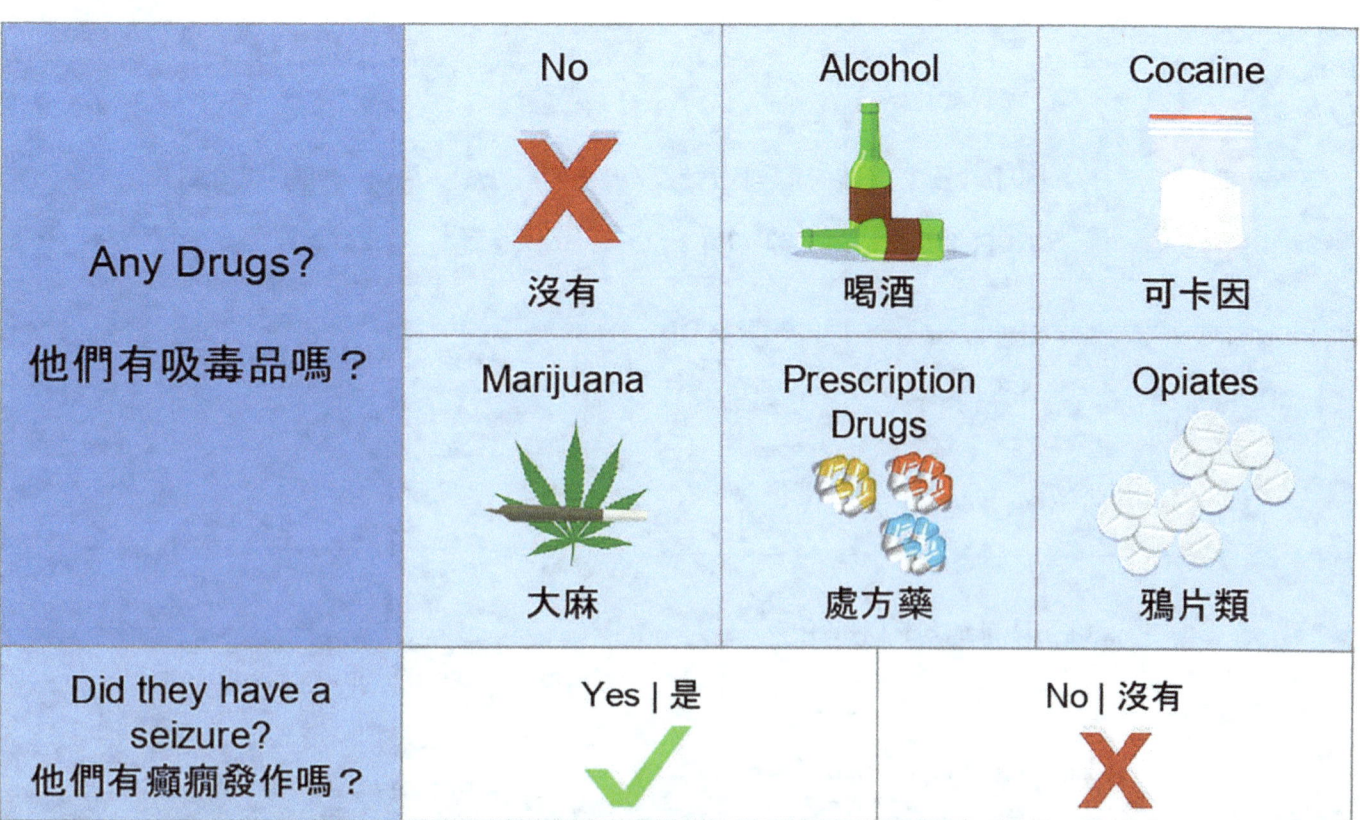

Any Drugs? 他們有吸毒品嗎?	No X 沒有	Alcohol 喝酒	Cocaine 可卡因
	Marijuana 大麻	Prescription Drugs 處方藥	Opiates 鴉片類

Did they have a seizure? 他們有癲癇發作嗎?	Yes | 是 ✔	No | 沒有 X

17

Headache/Dizziness

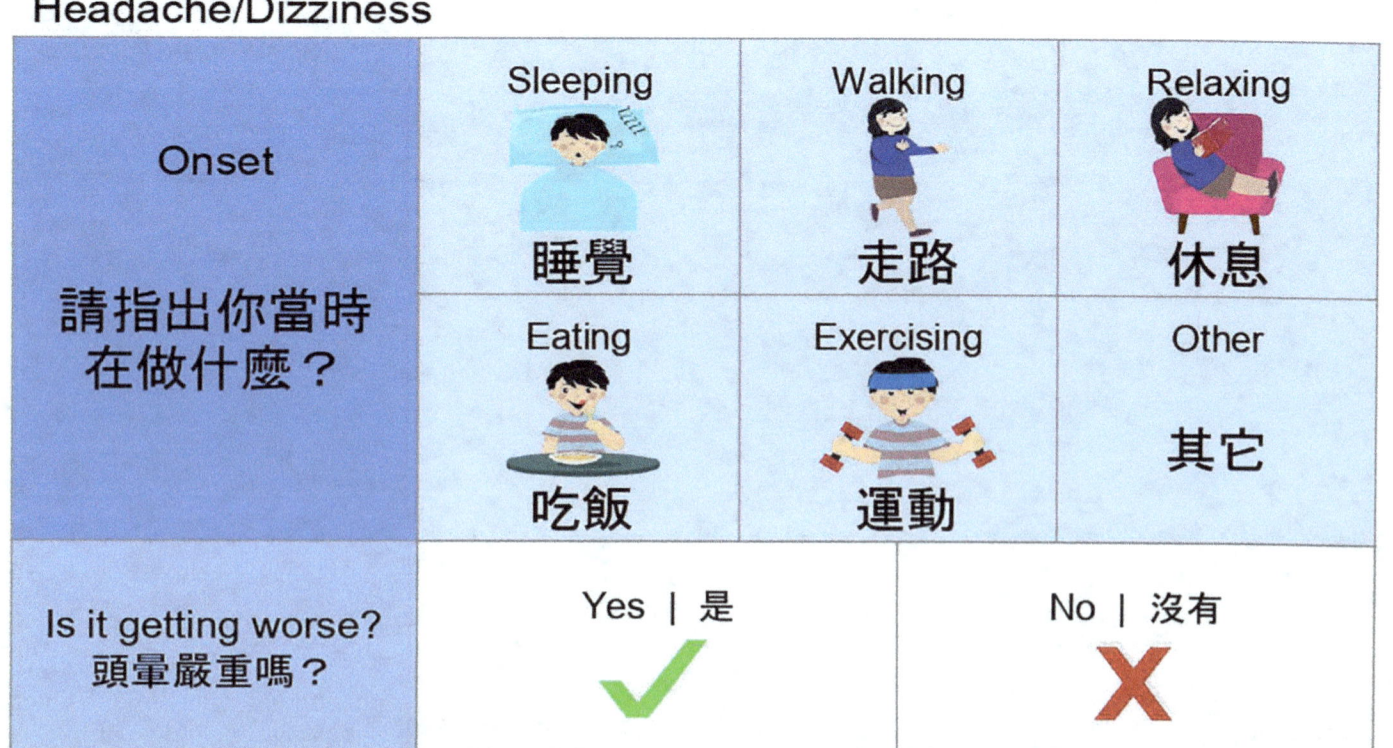

Onset 請指出你當時 在做什麼？	Sleeping 睡覺	Walking 走路	Relaxing 休息
	Eating 吃飯	Exercising 運動	Other 其它

Is it getting worse? 頭暈嚴重嗎？	Yes ｜ 是 ✓	No ｜ 沒有 ✗

Time 時間多久？	10 Mins 10分鐘	Half Hour 半小時	1 Hour 1小時
	2 Hours 2小時	3 Hours 3 小時	>4 Hours 4小時以上

Has this ever happened before? 以前發生過嗎？	Yes ｜ 有 ✔		No ｜ 沒有 ✘
Do you take your prescribed medications/您是否有服用醫生處方藥物？	Yes ｜ 是 ✔		No ｜ 沒有 ✘

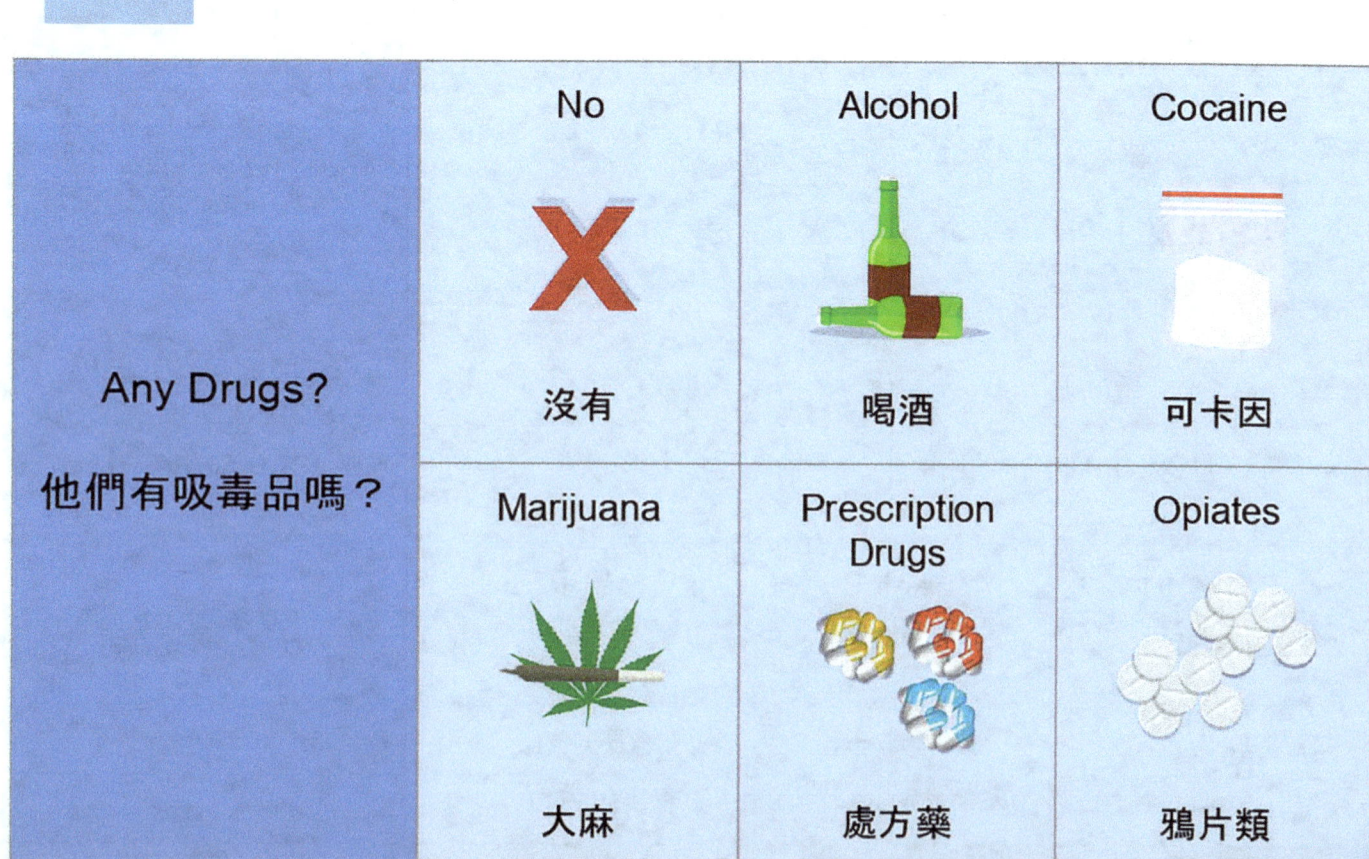

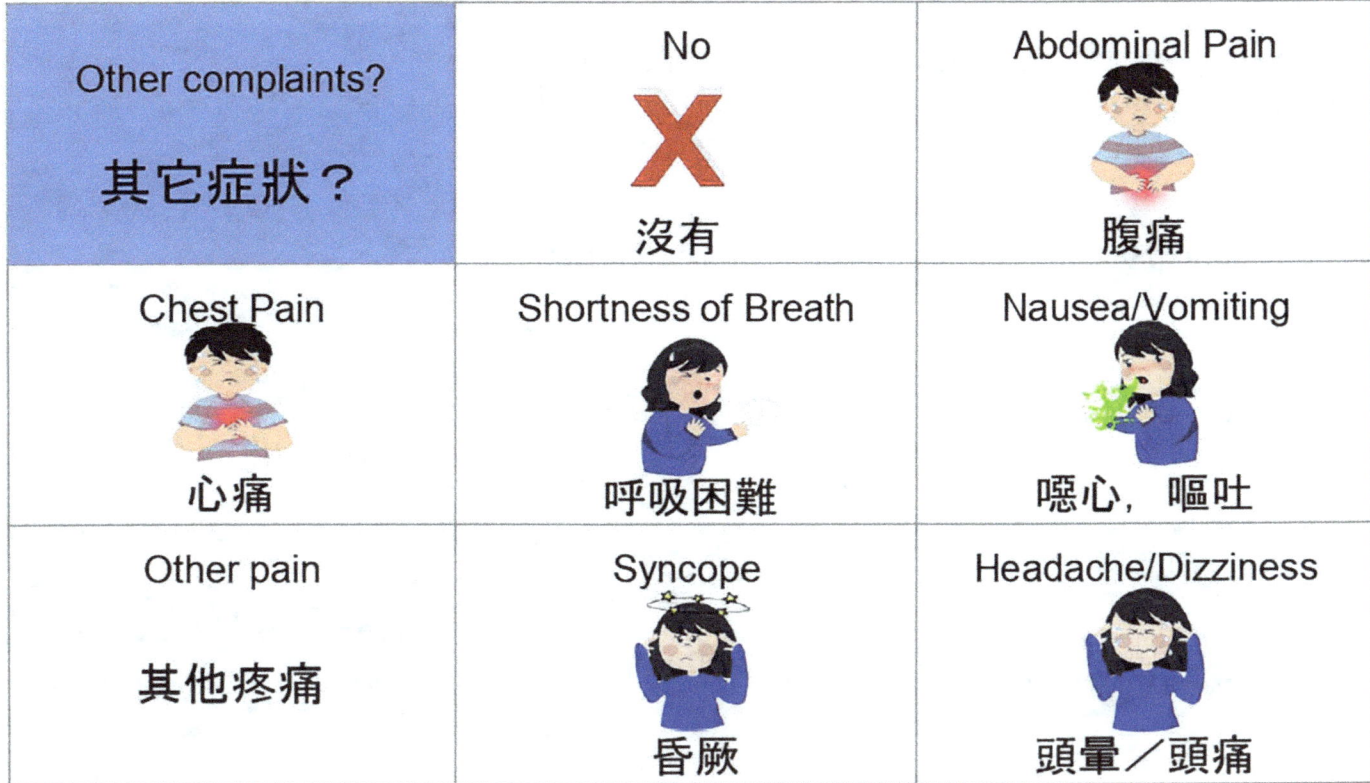

Other complaints? 其它症狀？	No **X** 沒有	Abdominal Pain 腹痛
Chest Pain 心痛	Shortness of Breath 呼吸困難	Nausea/Vomiting 噁心，嘔吐
Other pain 其他疼痛	Syncope 昏厥	Headache/Dizziness 頭暈／頭痛

Fall

Where are you hurting? 請指出你哪裡受傷？	No Injuries 沒有受傷		Can you point to where it hurts? 你能指出來嗎？
When did it happen? 時間多久？	10 Mins 10分鐘	Half Hour 半小時	1 Hour 1小時
	2 Hours 2小時	3 Hours 3 小時	>4 Hours 4小時以上
Did you lose consciousness? 當時有沒有失去知覺？	Yes | 有 For how long?多久？		No | 沒有 Are they behaving normal now?現在表現正常嗎？

Height of Fall?	1 Feet 1英尺	2-3 Feet 2-3英尺	4-5 Feet 4-5 英尺
由多高摔下來？	6-10 Feet 6-10 英尺	11-15 Feet 11-15 英尺	>20 Feet 20英尺以上
Why did you fall? 你是什麼原因摔倒？	Trip & Fall/ Rolled out of Bed 滑倒／下床滑倒		Weakness/ Dizziness 虛弱／頭暈
	Fainting/Syncope 昏厥		Other Reason 其他原因
Are you on any blood thinning medications? 你有服用溶血藥物嗎？	Yes/有 Can we see the medications/我們可以看藥物嗎？		No/沒有 Can we see the medications/我們可以看藥物嗎？

Trauma

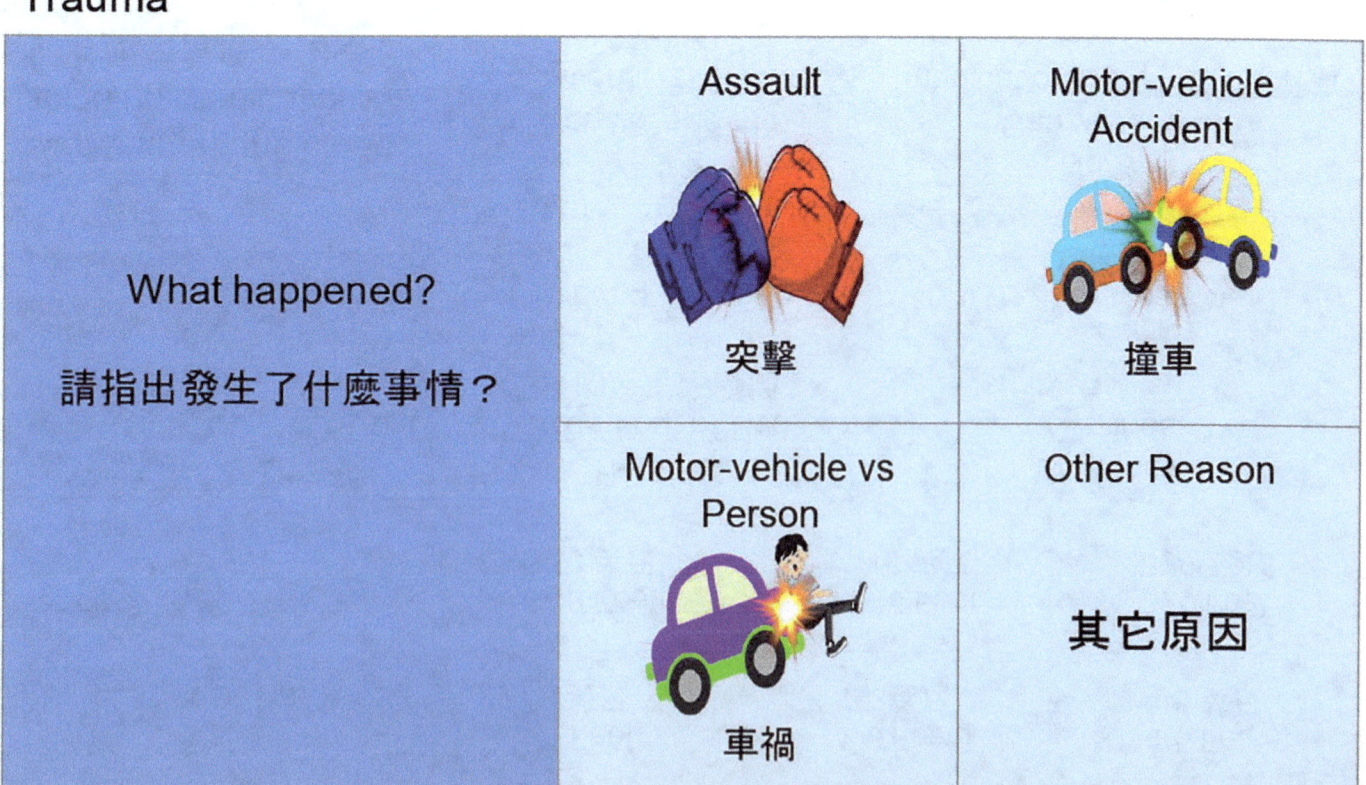

What happened?

請指出發生了什麼事情？

Assault
突擊

Motor-vehicle Accident
撞車

Motor-vehicle vs Person
車禍

Other Reason
其它原因

Where are you hurting? 你在哪裡受傷?	No Injuries 沒有受傷	Can you point to where it hurts? 你能指出?
When did it happen? 時間多久?	10 Mins 10分鐘	Half Hour 半小時	1 Hour 1小時
	2 Hours 2小時	3 Hours 3 小時	>4 Hours 4小時以上
Speed of Vehicle/ 當時車速?	5-10 MPH 5-10英里每小時	10-15 MPH 10-15英里每小時	15-20 MPH 15-20英里每小時
	20-30 MPH 20-30英里每小時	30-40 MPH 30-40英里每小時	Above 50 MPH 50英里每小時以上

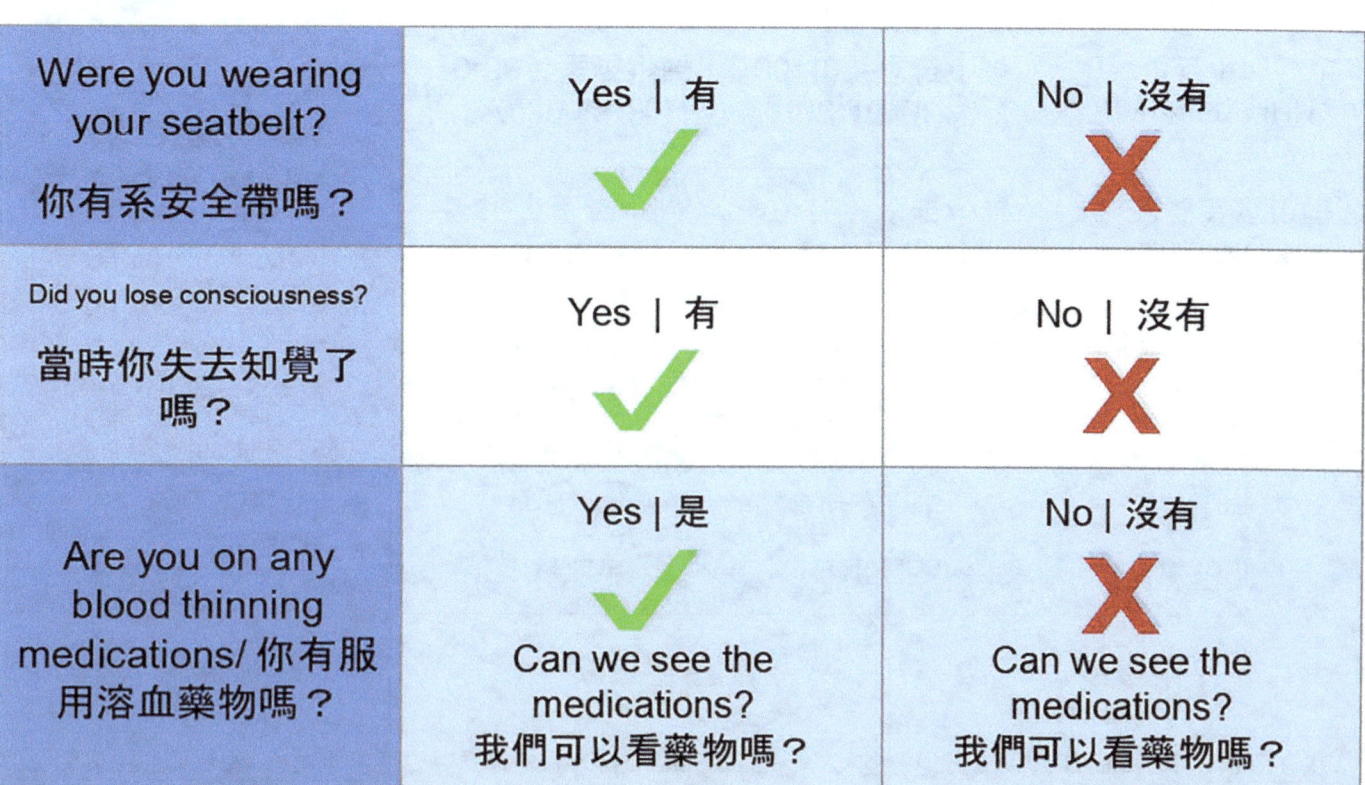

Miscellaneous Questions

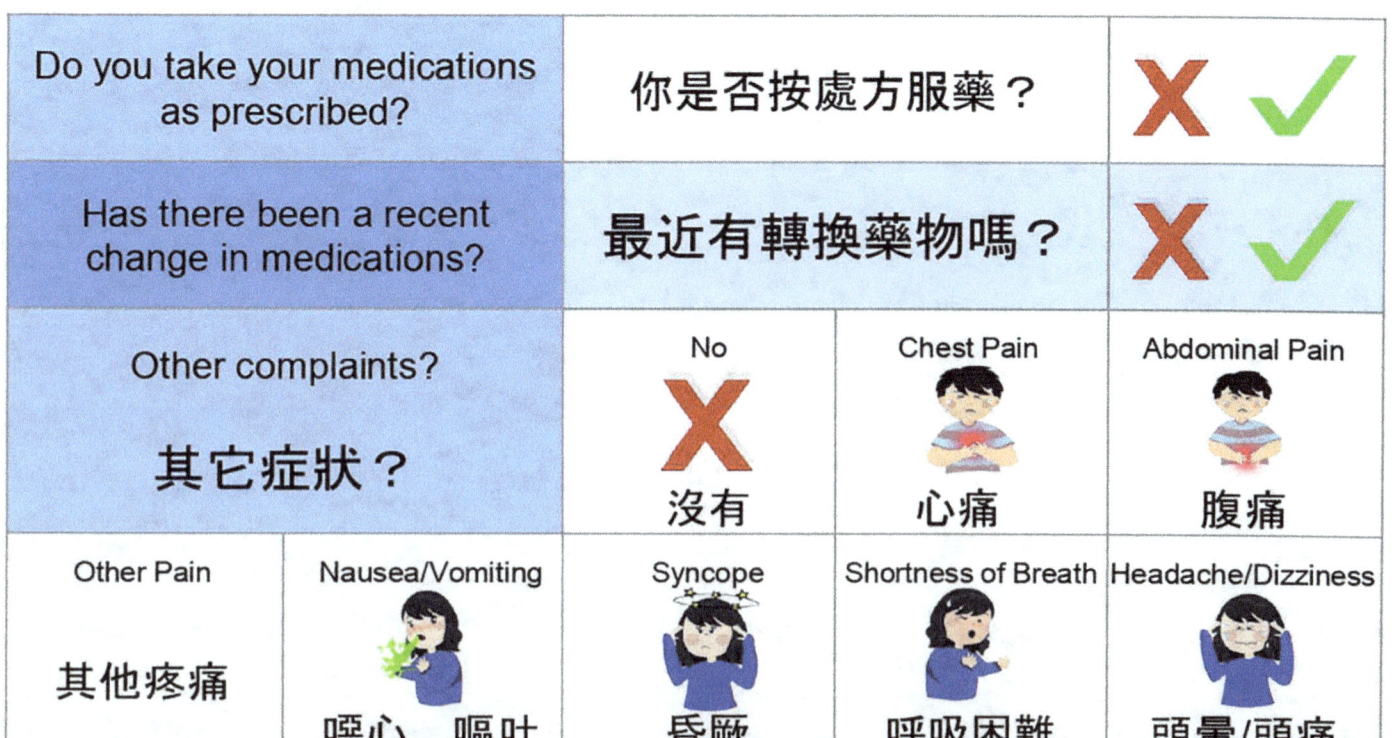

Do you take your medications as prescribed?	你是否按處方服藥？	X ✓
Has there been a recent change in medications?	最近有轉換藥物嗎？	X ✓

Other complaints?

其它症狀？

No	Chest Pain	Abdominal Pain
X		
沒有	心痛	腹痛

Other Pain	Nausea/Vomiting	Syncope	Shortness of Breath	Headache/Dizziness
其他疼痛	噁心，嘔吐	昏厥	呼吸困難	頭暈/頭痛

When was the last time you ate something? 你上一次吃飯是什麼時候?	10 Mins 10 分鐘	Half Hour 半小時	1 Hour 1 小時
	2 Hour 2 小時	3 Hour 3 小時	>4 Hours 4 小時以上
Have you ever felt this way before?	你曾經有過這種感覺嗎?		X ✓
Does the patient have a DNR order?Can we see it?	患者是否不要救治?可以看嗎?		X ✓
Do you want to go to the hospital?	你要去醫院嗎?		X ✓

23

Medical History - 病史.請指出

Asthma	哮喘
Atrial Fibrillation	心跳異常
Cancer	癌症
COPD	慢性阻塞型肺炎
Diabetes	糖尿病
Hypertension	高血壓
Heart Failure	心臟衰竭

Liver Problems	肝病
Myocardial Infarctions	心髒病
Renal Problems	腎臟疾病
Seizures	癲癇
Stroke	中風

24

Medications - 服用藥物.請指出

Aspirin	阿斯匹林
Atorvastatin	阿脫伐他酊
Benadryl	貝納德里
Blood Thinners	血液稀釋劑
Erythromycin	紅霉素
Fentanyl	芬太尼
Insulin	胰島素

Ketamine	氯胺酮
Metformin	二甲雙胍
Metoprolol	美托洛爾
Morphine	嗎啡
Penicillin	青霉素
Sulfa Drugs	磺胺藥
Warfarin	華法林

Allergies - 過敏藥物.請指出

No Known Drug Allergies	沒有藥物過敏
Aspirin	阿司匹林
Atorvastatin	阿托伐他汀
Benadryl	貝納德里
Blood Thinners	血液稀釋劑
Erythromycin	紅霉素
Fentanyl	芬太尼

Ketamine	氯胺酮
Metformin	二甲雙胍
Metoprolol	美托洛爾
Morphine	嗎啡
Penicillin	青霉素
Sulfa Drugs	磺胺藥
Warfarin	華法林

Intervention Phrases

I am going to start a IV on you	我將要給你靜脈注射
I am going to check your blood sugar	我將要給你測試血糖
I am going to put a collar around your neck	我要給你戴上頸托
I am going to assess your heart, these stickers are going to be on your left chest	我要評估你的心跳，將貼紙貼在你的左胸部

I am going to give you a medication. Let me know if your symptoms get better or worst	我要給你服藥，判斷你的症狀好轉／惡化		
How are you feeling now? 你現在疼痛的程度如何？	**0** 	**2** 	**4**
	6 	**8** 	**10**

27

Español

Spanish

Hello I am a medical professional. I do not speak your language, but I will be using this translation guide to help me. Please read the question and point to the correct choice

Hola! Soy un profesional médico. No hablo español, pero voy a usar esta guía de traducción para ayudarme. Por favor, lea la pregunta y señale la opción correcta

Alert & Oriented Questions

What is your name?		¿Cómo se llama?	
Where are we now? **¿Dónde se encuentra ahora?**	House En su Casa	Restaurant Restaurante	Outside En El Exterior
	Store Tienda	Ambulance Ambulancia	Other Otro lugar

	Morning	Afternoon	Evening
What time of day is it? **¿Qué momento del día es?**	Mañana	Tarde	Noche
Who are we?	Mom Madre	Chef Cocinero/a	Farmer Granjero/a
¿Quién soy?	Paramedic Paramédico	Dad Padre	Construction Worker Obrero

29

Chief Complaints

What's going on today?	¿Qué lo aqueja hoy? Elija a continuación
Chest Pain | p.31-32 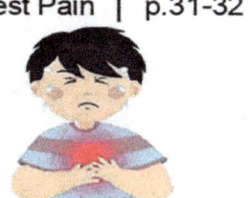 **Dolor de Pecho**	Abdominal Pain | p.33-34 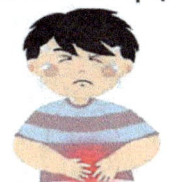 **Dolor Abdominal**
Other Pains | p.35-36 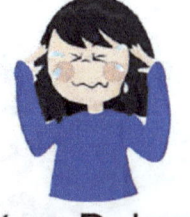 **Otros Dolores**	Breathing Problem | p.37-38 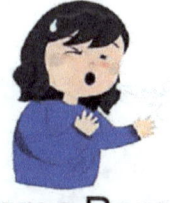 **Problema Respiratorio**

Nausea/Vomiting | p.39-40 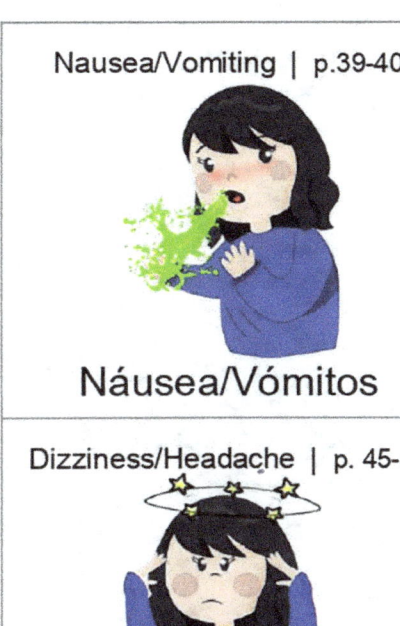 Náusea/Vómitos	Syncope | p. 41-42 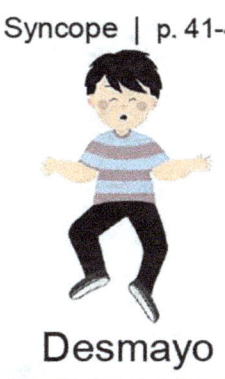 Desmayo	ALOC/Stroke | p. 43-44 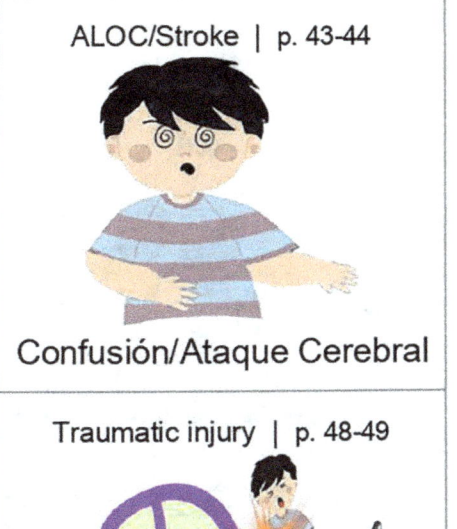 Confusión/Ataque Cerebral
Dizziness/Headache | p. 45-46 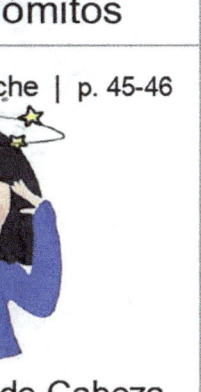 Mareos/Dolor de Cabeza	Fall | p. 47 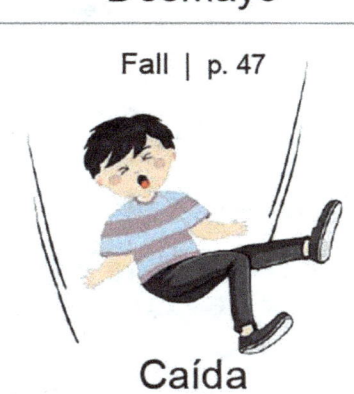 Caída	Traumatic injury | p. 48-49 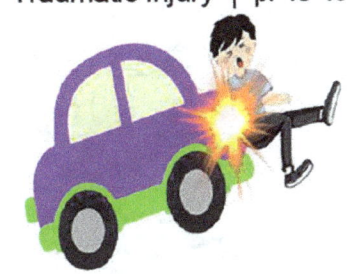 Traumatismo distinto a caída

Chest Pain/Dolor de Pecho

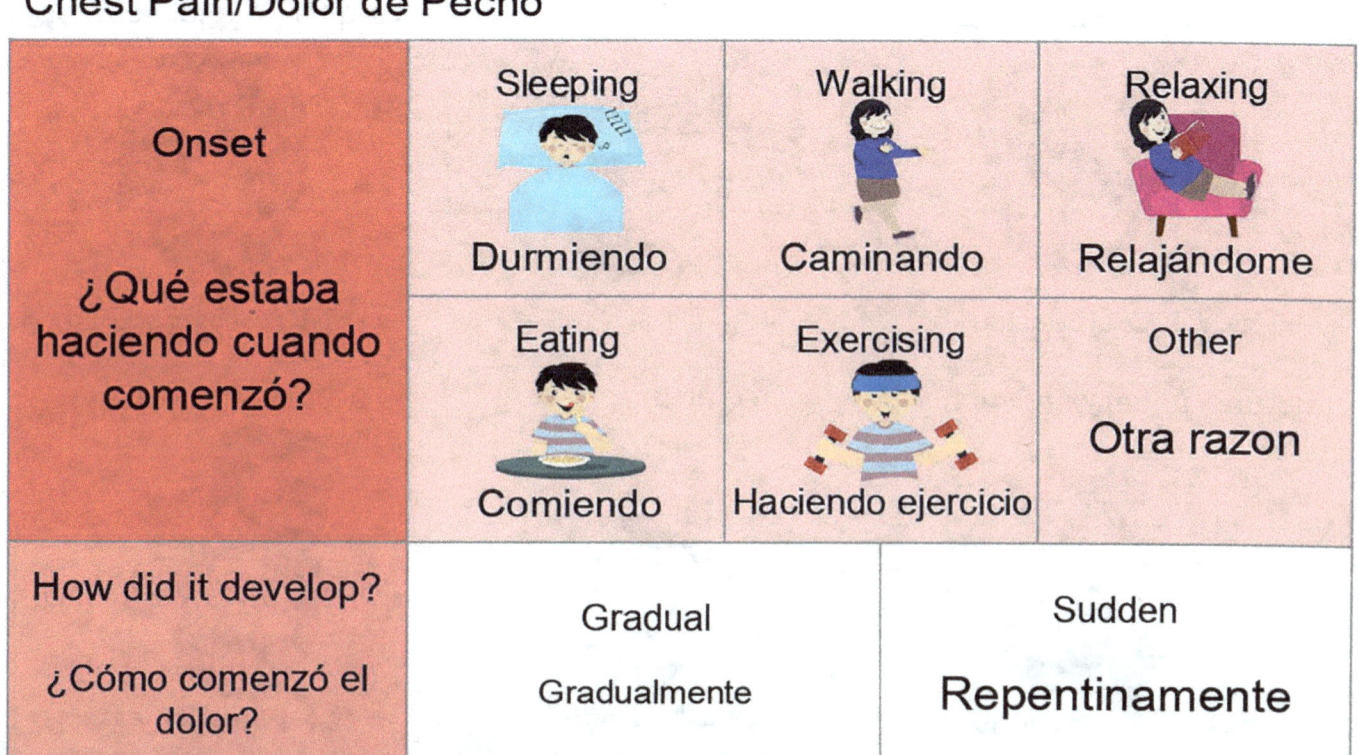

Onset ¿Qué estaba haciendo cuando comenzó?	Sleeping Durmiendo	Walking Caminando	Relaxing Relajándome
	Eating Comiendo	Exercising Haciendo ejercicio	Other Otra razon
How did it develop? ¿Cómo comenzó el dolor?	Gradual Gradualmente		Sudden Repentinamente

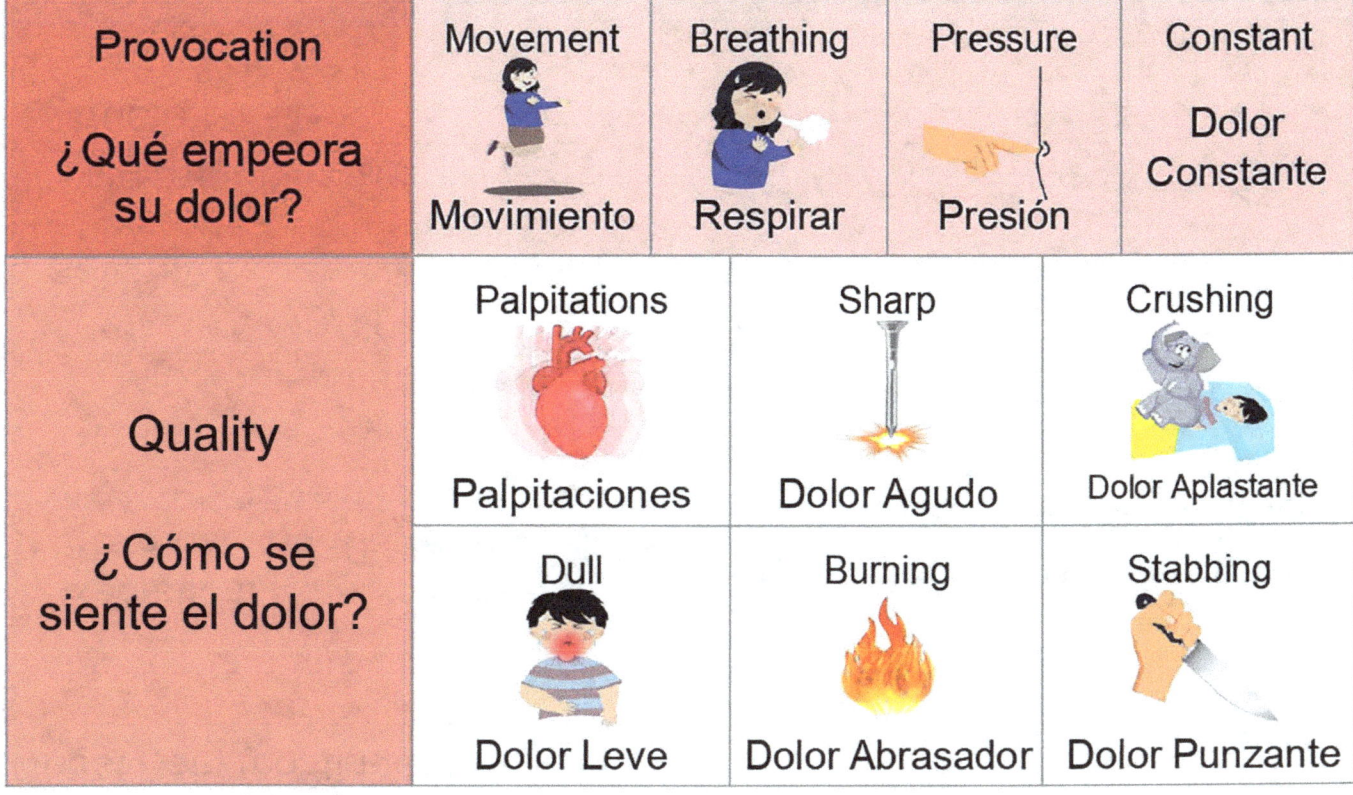

Provocation ¿Qué empeora su dolor?	Movement Movimiento	Breathing Respirar	Pressure Presión	Constant Dolor Constante
Quality ¿Cómo se siente el dolor?	Palpitations Palpitaciones	Sharp Dolor Agudo		Crushing Dolor Aplastante
	Dull Dolor Leve	Burning Dolor Abrasador		Stabbing Dolor Punzante

31

Chest Pain (continued)

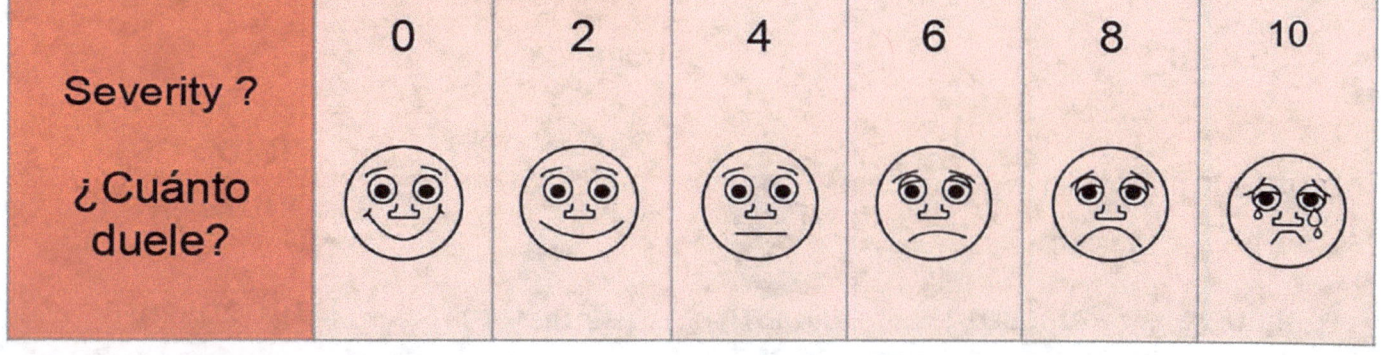

| Radiation: Point to where it hurts most and where the pain travels to | Señale dónde más le duele y hacia donde viaja el dolor |

Time ¿A qué hora comenzaron sus síntomas?	10 Mins 10 Minutos	Half Hour Media Hora	1 Hour 1 Hora
	2 Hours 2 Horas	3 Hours 3 Horas	>4 Hours 4 Horas

Pertinent Negatives: Are you having any of the following ¿Tiene algunas de las siguientes afecciones médicas?	No **X**	Abdominal Pain Dolor Abdominal	Breathing Difficulty Problema Respiratorio
		Nausea/Vomiting Náusea y Vómitos	Other Pains Otro Dolor

32

Abdominal Pain

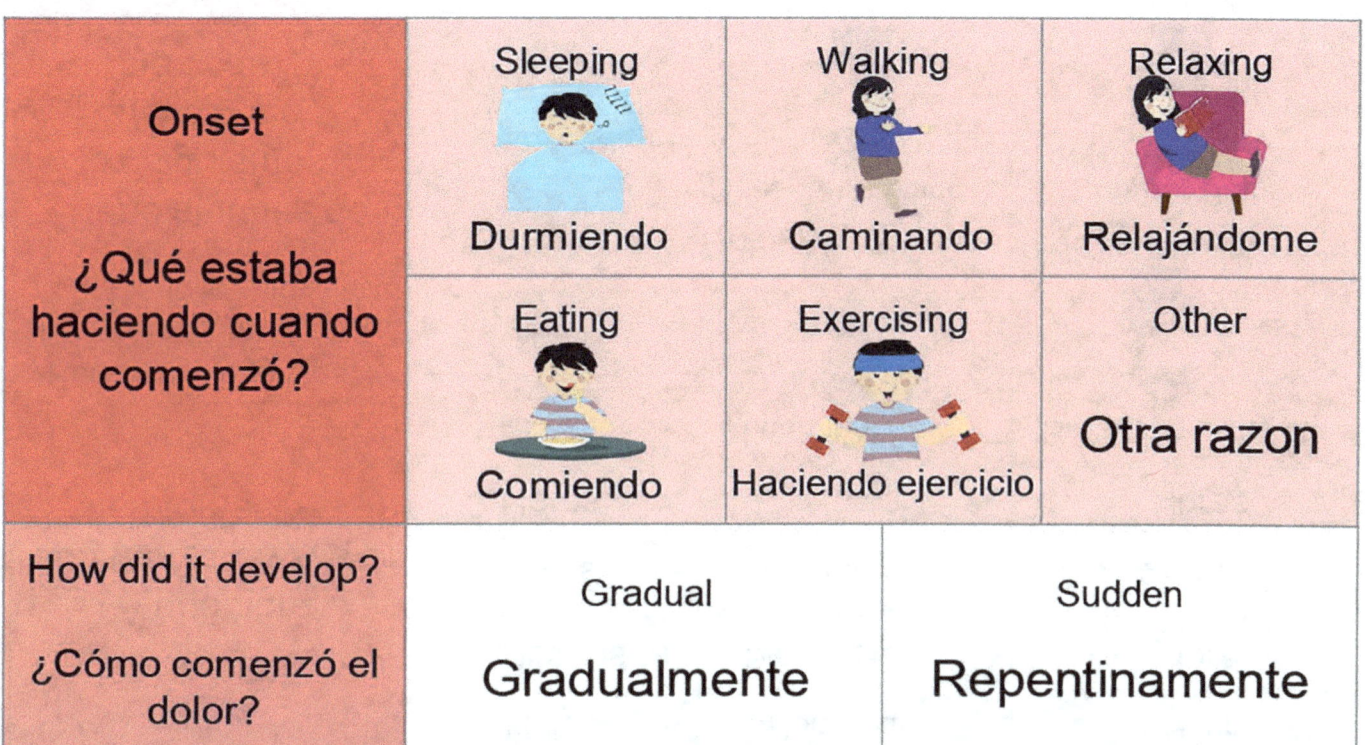

Onset ¿Qué estaba haciendo cuando comenzó?	Sleeping Durmiendo	Walking Caminando	Relaxing Relajándome
	Eating Comiendo	Exercising Haciendo ejercicio	Other Otra razon
How did it develop? ¿Cómo comenzó el dolor?	Gradual Gradualmente		Sudden Repentinamente

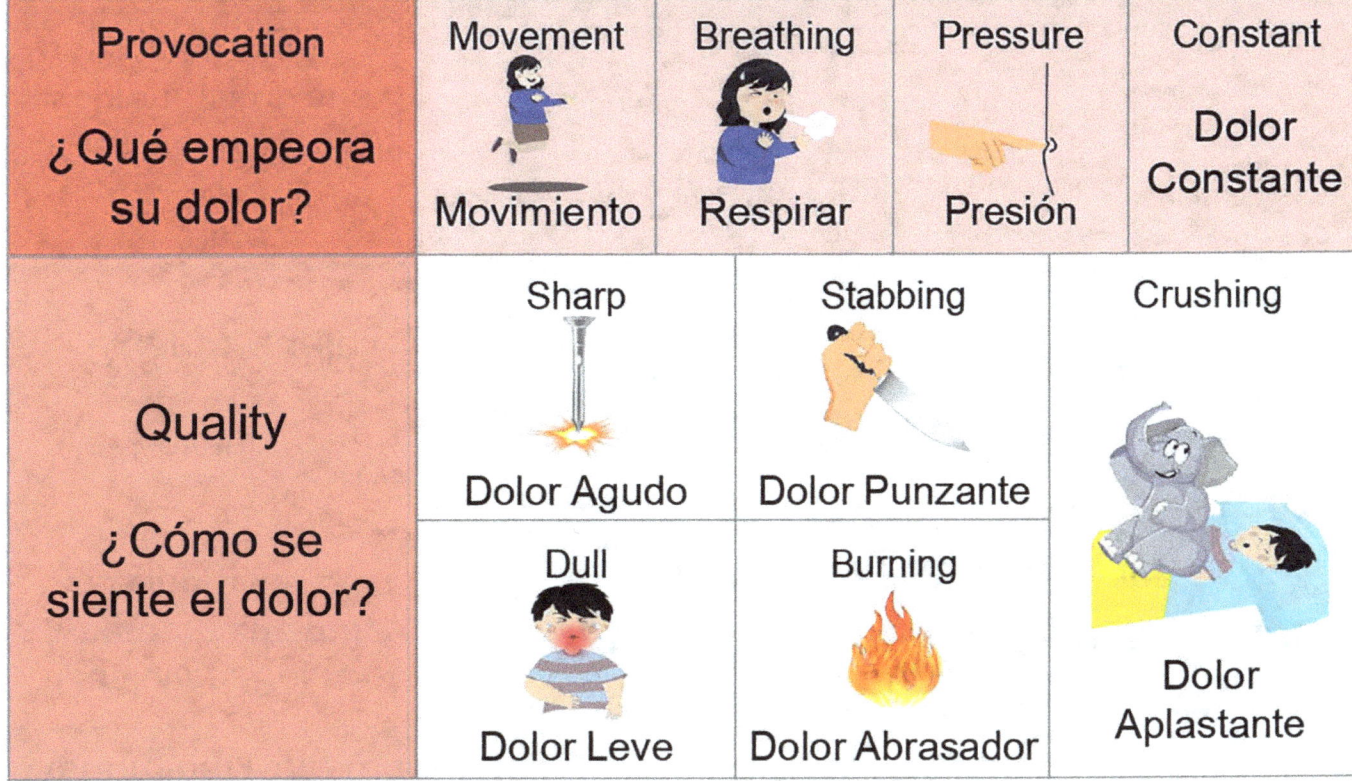

Provocation ¿Qué empeora su dolor?	Movement Movimiento	Breathing Respirar	Pressure Presión	Constant Dolor Constante
Quality ¿Cómo se siente el dolor?	Sharp Dolor Agudo	Stabbing Dolor Punzante	Crushing Dolor Aplastante	
	Dull Dolor Leve	Burning Dolor Abrasador		

Abdominal Pain (continued)

Radiation: Point to where it hurts most and where the pain travels to	Señale dónde más le duele y hacia donde viaja el dolor					
Severity ? ¿Cuánto duele?	0	2	4	6	8	10
Time ¿A qué hora comenzaron sus síntomas?	10 Mins 10 Minutos		Half Hour Media Hora		1 Hour 1 Hora	
	2 Hours 2 Horas		3 Hours 3 Horas		>4 Hours Más de 4 Horas	

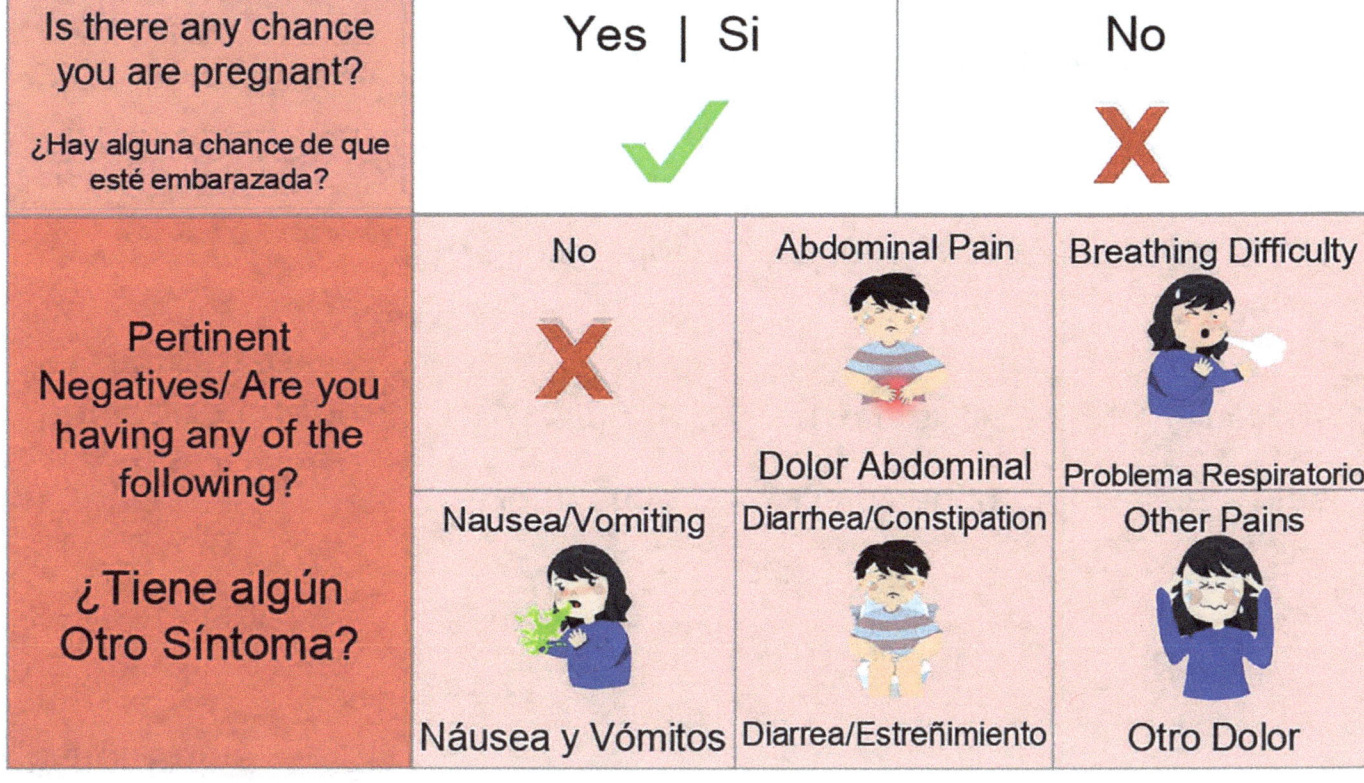

Is there any chance you are pregnant? ¿Hay alguna chance de que esté embarazada?	Yes | Si ✔	No X	
Pertinent Negatives/ Are you having any of the following? ¿Tiene algún Otro Síntoma?	No X	Abdominal Pain Dolor Abdominal	Breathing Difficulty Problema Respiratorio
	Nausea/Vomiting Náusea y Vómitos	Diarrhea/Constipation Diarrea/Estreñimiento	Other Pains Otro Dolor

34

Other Pains

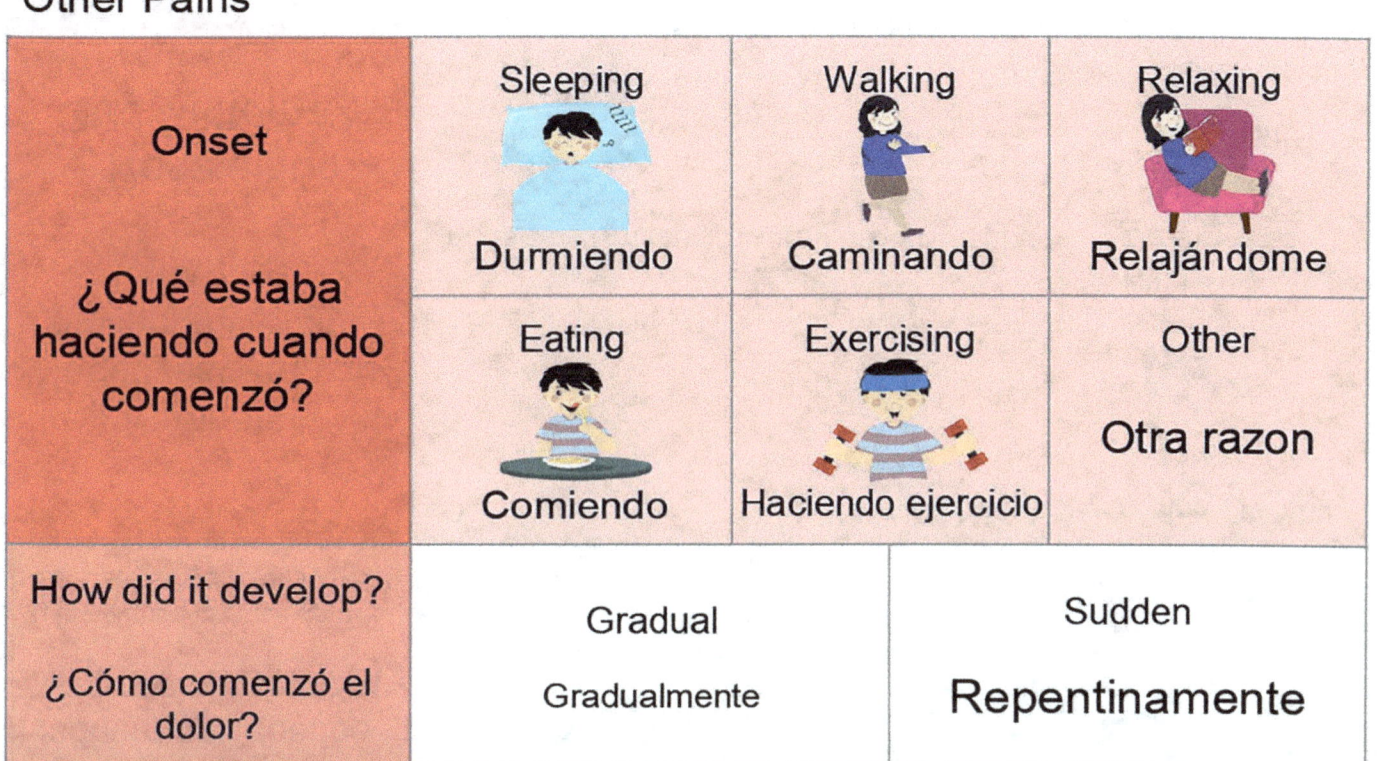

Onset ¿Qué estaba haciendo cuando comenzó?	Sleeping Durmiendo	Walking Caminando	Relaxing Relajándome
	Eating Comiendo	Exercising Haciendo ejercicio	Other Otra razon
How did it develop? ¿Cómo comenzó el dolor?	Gradual Gradualmente		Sudden Repentinamente

Provocation ¿Qué empeora su dolor?	Movement 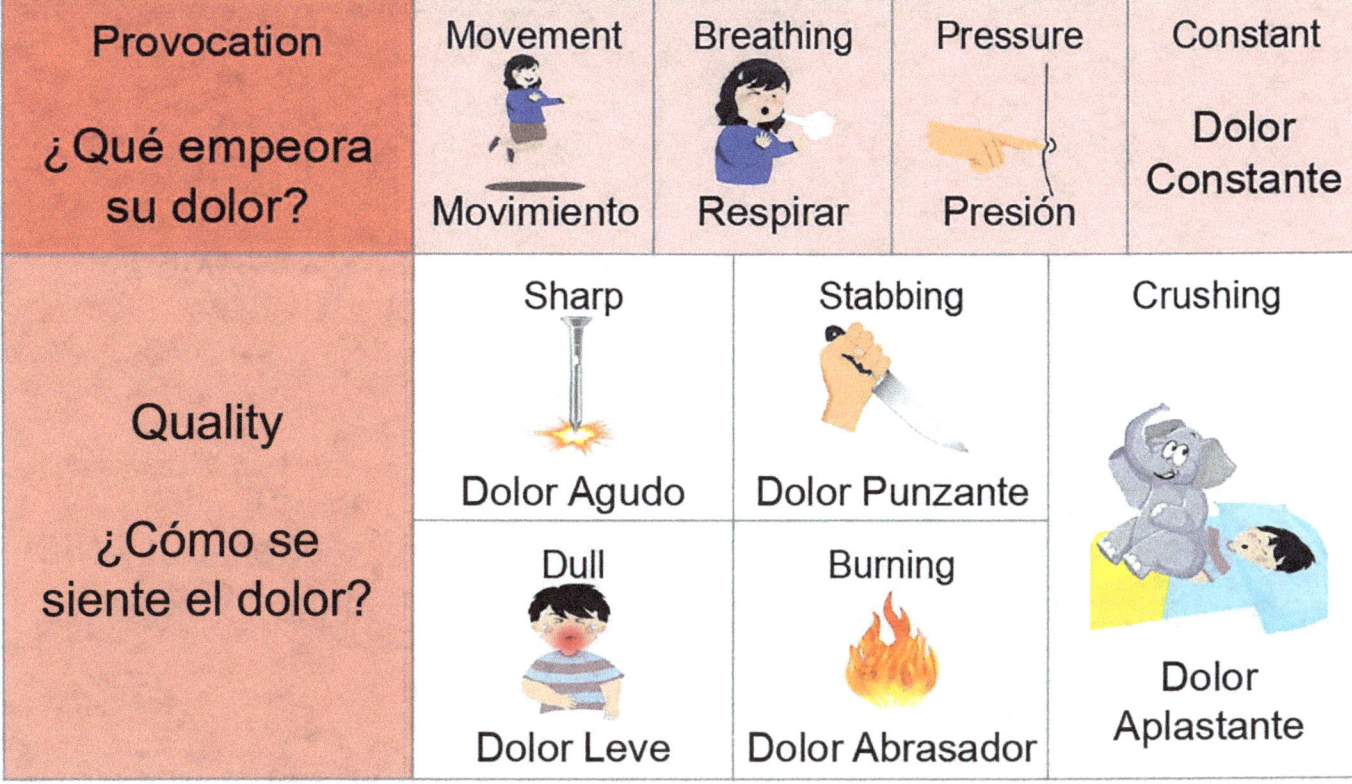Movimiento	Breathing Respirar	Pressure Presión	Constant Dolor Constante
Quality ¿Cómo se siente el dolor?	Sharp Dolor Agudo Dull Dolor Leve	Stabbing Dolor Punzante Burning Dolor Abrasador		Crushing Dolor Aplastante

35

Other Pains (continued)

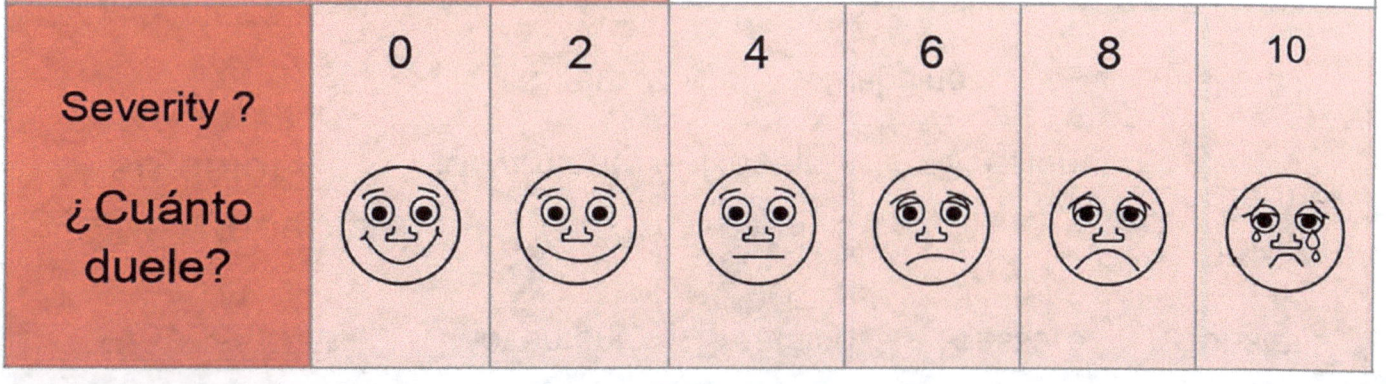

Radiation: Point to where it hurts most and where the pain travels to	Radiación: Señale dónde más le duele y hacia donde viaja el dolor					
Severity ? ¿Cuánto duele?	0	2	4	6	8	10

Time ¿A qué hora comenzaron sus síntomas?	10 Mins 10 Minutos	Half Hour Media Hora	1 Hour 1 Hora
	2 Hours 2 Horas	3 Hours 3 Horas	>4 Hours Mas de 4 Horas
Pertinent Negatives/ Are you having any of the following? ¿Algún Otro Síntoma?	No X	Abdominal Pain Dolor Abdominal	Breathing Difficulty Problema Respiratorio
	Nausea/Vomiting Náusea y Vómitos	Diarrhea/Constipation Diarrea/Estreñimiento	Other Pains Otro Dolor

36

Shortness of Breath

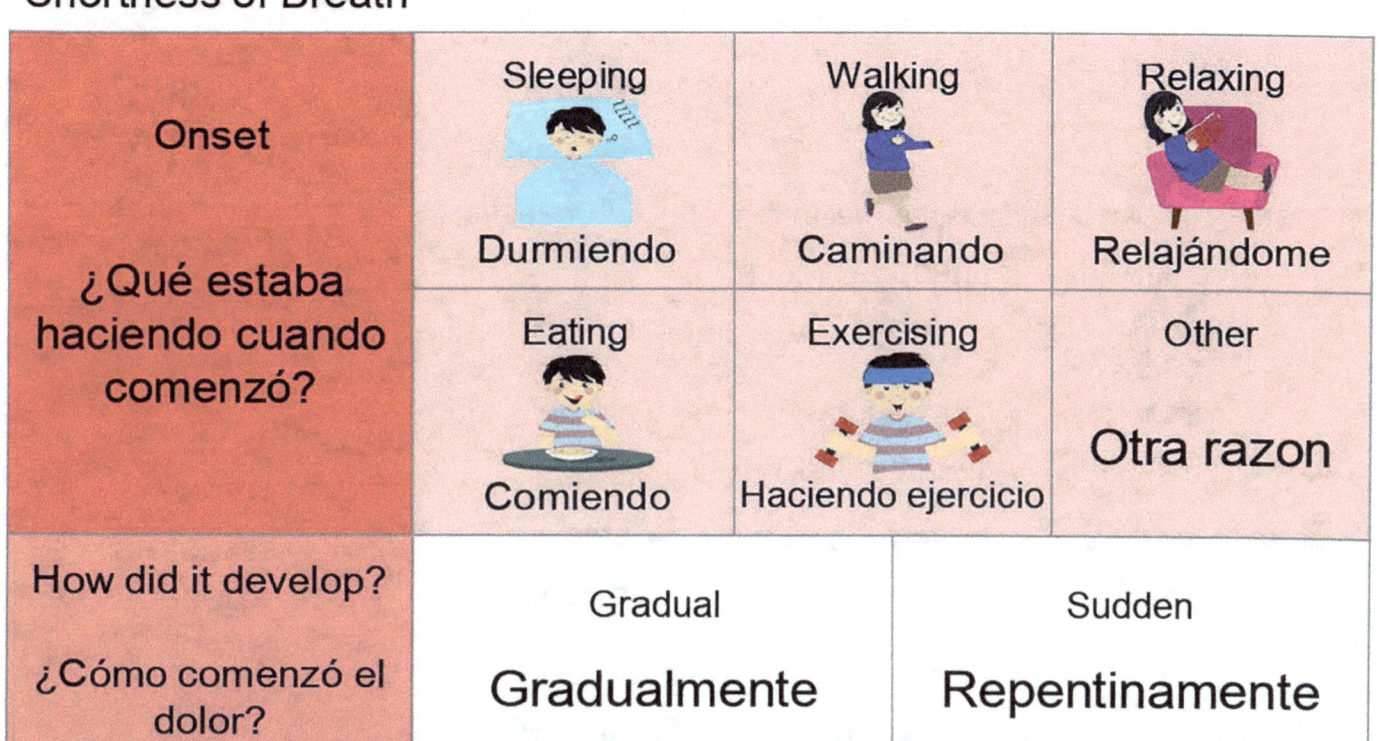

Onset ¿Qué estaba haciendo cuando comenzó?	Sleeping Durmiendo	Walking Caminando	Relaxing Relajándome
	Eating Comiendo	Exercising Haciendo ejercicio	Other Otra razon

How did it develop? ¿Cómo comenzó el dolor?	Gradual Gradualmente	Sudden Repentinamente

Do you have associated chest pain? Dolor de Pecho Asociado	Yes | Si 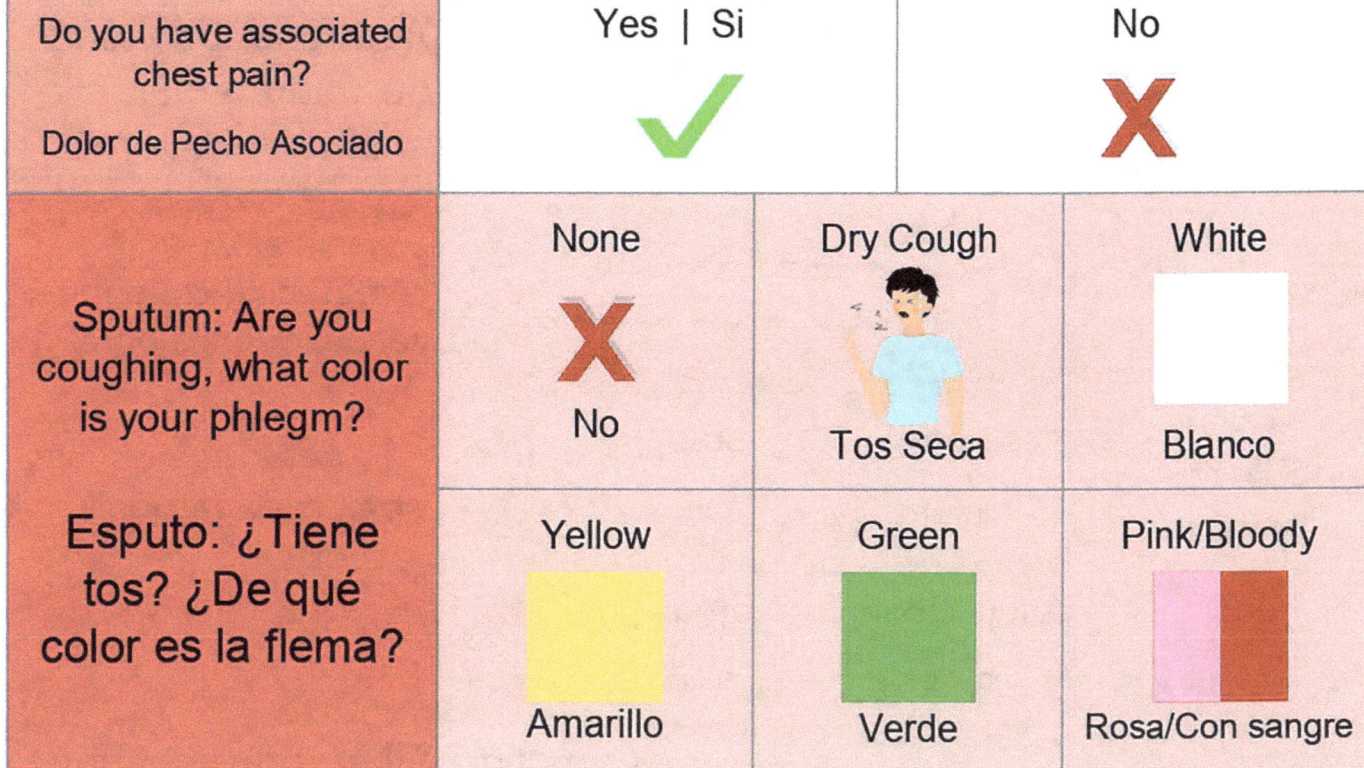		No X	
Sputum: Are you coughing, what color is your phlegm? Esputo: ¿Tiene tos? ¿De qué color es la flema?	None X No	Dry Cough Tos Seca	White Blanco	
	Yellow Amarillo	Green Verde	Pink/Bloody Rosa/Con sangre	

37

Shortness of Breath (continued)

Time ¿A qué hora comenzaron sus síntomas?	10 Mins 10 Minutos	Half Hour Media Hora	1 Hour 1 Hora
	2 Hours 2 Horas	3 Hours 3 Horas	>4 Hours Más de 4 Horas
Exertion: Does movement and exercise make it worse? ¿El movimiento y el ejercicio empeoran su dificultad respiratoria?	Yes | Si ✔		No ✗

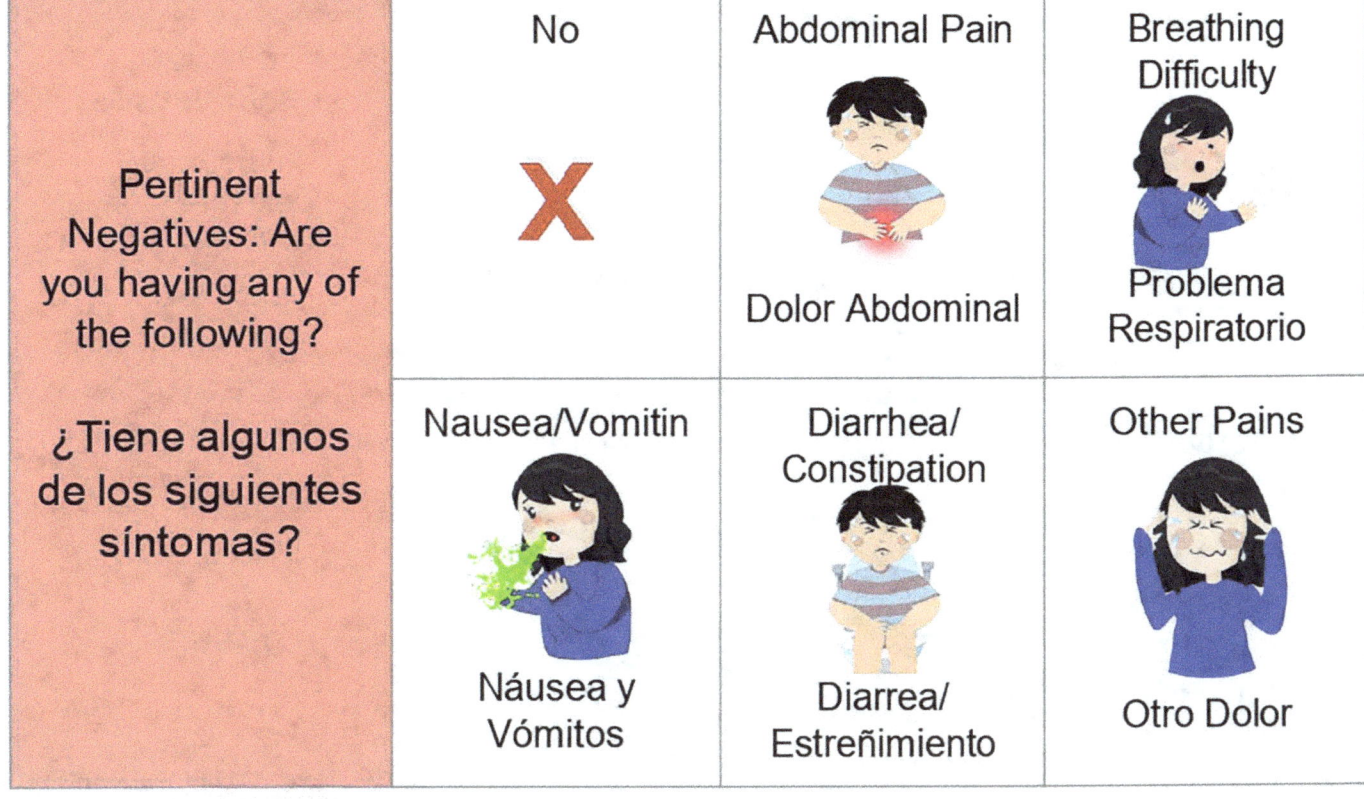

Pertinent Negatives: Are you having any of the following? ¿Tiene algunos de los siguientes síntomas?	No X	Abdominal Pain Dolor Abdominal	Breathing Difficulty Problema Respiratorio
	Nausea/Vomitin Náusea y Vómitos	Diarrhea/ Constipation Diarrea/ Estreñimiento	Other Pains Otro Dolor

Nausea and Vomiting

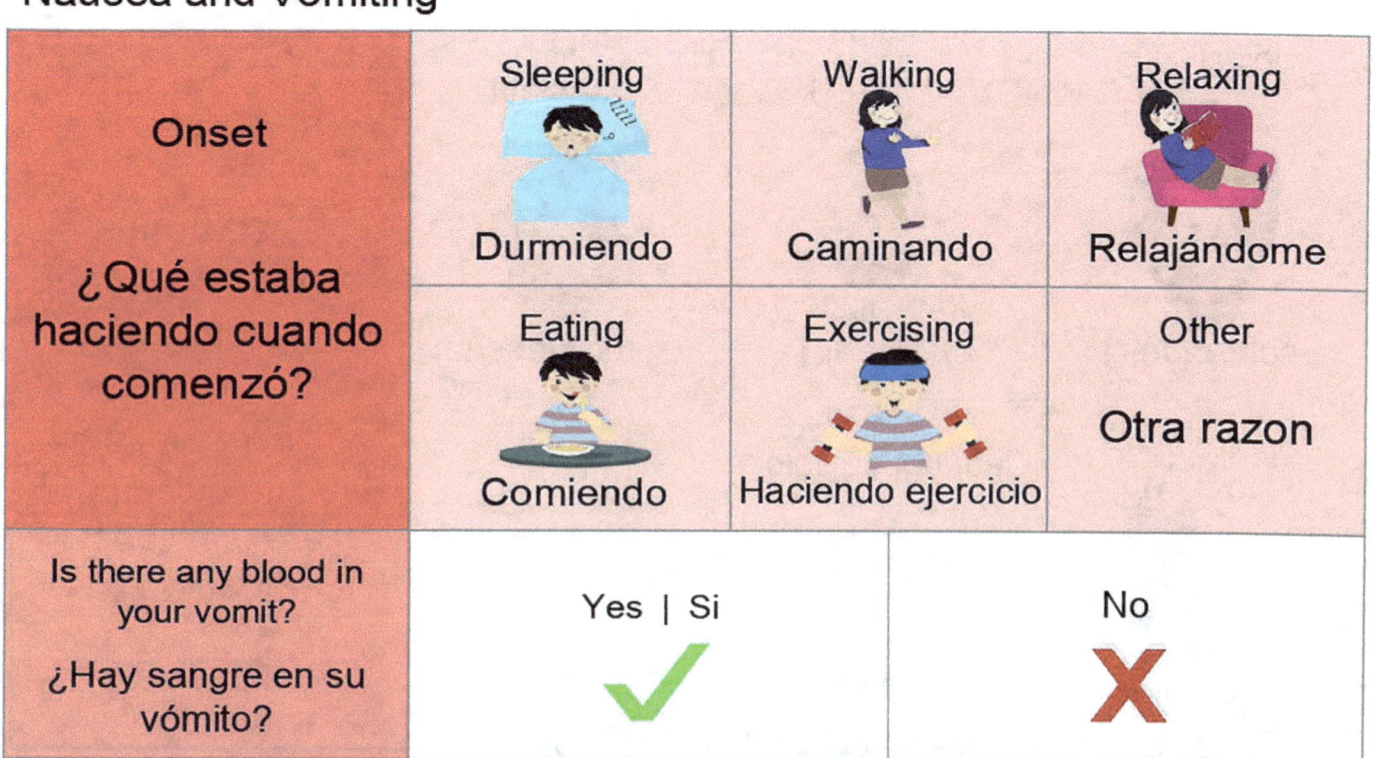

Onset ¿Qué estaba haciendo cuando comenzó?	Sleeping Durmiendo	Walking Caminando	Relaxing Relajándome
	Eating Comiendo	Exercising Haciendo ejercicio	Other Otra razon
Is there any blood in your vomit? ¿Hay sangre en su vómito?	Yes | Si ✔		No ✖

Time ¿A qué hora comenzaron sus síntomas?	10 Mins 10 Minutos	Half Hour Media Hora	1 Hour 1 Hora
	2 Hours 2 Horas	3 Hours 3 Horas	>4 Hours Más de 4 Horas
Are you having abdominal pain? ¿Tiene dolor abdominal?	Yes | Si ✅		No ❌
Are you pregnant? ¿Está embarazada?	Yes | Si ✅ How many months? ¿De cuántos meses está su embarazo?		No ❌

39

Nausea and Vomiting (continued)

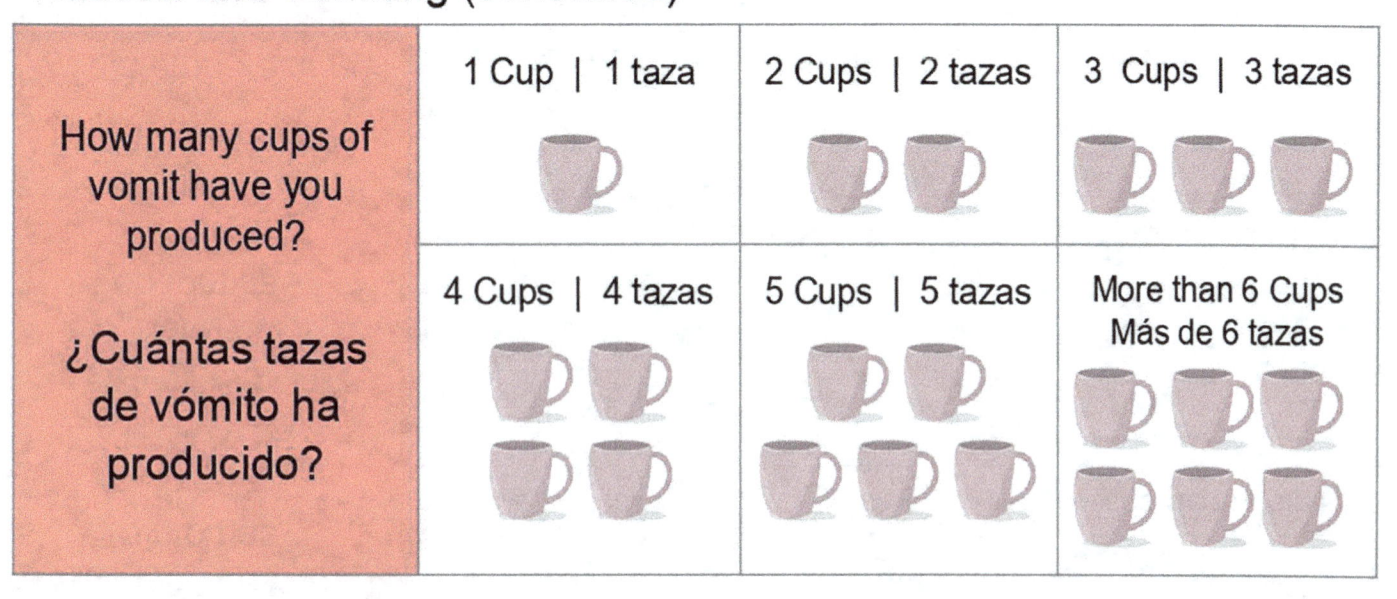

How many cups of vomit have you produced? ¿Cuántas tazas de vómito ha producido?	1 Cup | 1 taza	2 Cups | 2 tazas	3 Cups | 3 tazas
	4 Cups | 4 tazas	5 Cups | 5 tazas	More than 6 Cups Más de 6 tazas

Pertinent Negatives: Are you having any of the following? ¿Tiene algunos de los siguientes síntomas?	No X	Abdominal Pain Dolor Abdominal	Breathing Difficulty Problema Respiratorio
	Nausea/Vomitin Náusea y Vómitos	Diarrhea/ Constipation Diarrea/ Estreñimiento	Other Pains Otro Dolor

40

Syncope

Onset ¿Qué estaba haciendo cuando comenzó?	Sleeping Durmiendo	Walking Caminando	Relaxing Relajándome
	Eating Comiendo	Exercising Haciendo ejercicio	Other Otra razon
Did you suffer any injuries? ¿Sufrió alguna lesión?	No X	Can you point to where it hurts? ¿Puede señalar dónde le duele?	

Time ¿A qué hora comenzaron sus síntomas?	10 Mins 10 Minutos	Half Hour Media Hora	1 Hour 1 Hora
	2 Hours 2 Horas	3 Hours 3 Horas	>4 Hours Mas de 4 Horas
What symptoms did you have prior? ¿Qué síntomas tuvo previamente?	Felt Fine Me sentí bien	Abdominal Pain Dolor Abdominal	Chest Pain Dolor de Pecho
	Nausea/Vomiting Náusea y Vómitos	Shortness of Breath Problema Respiratorio	Dizziness/Headache Mareos/Dolor de Cabeza

41

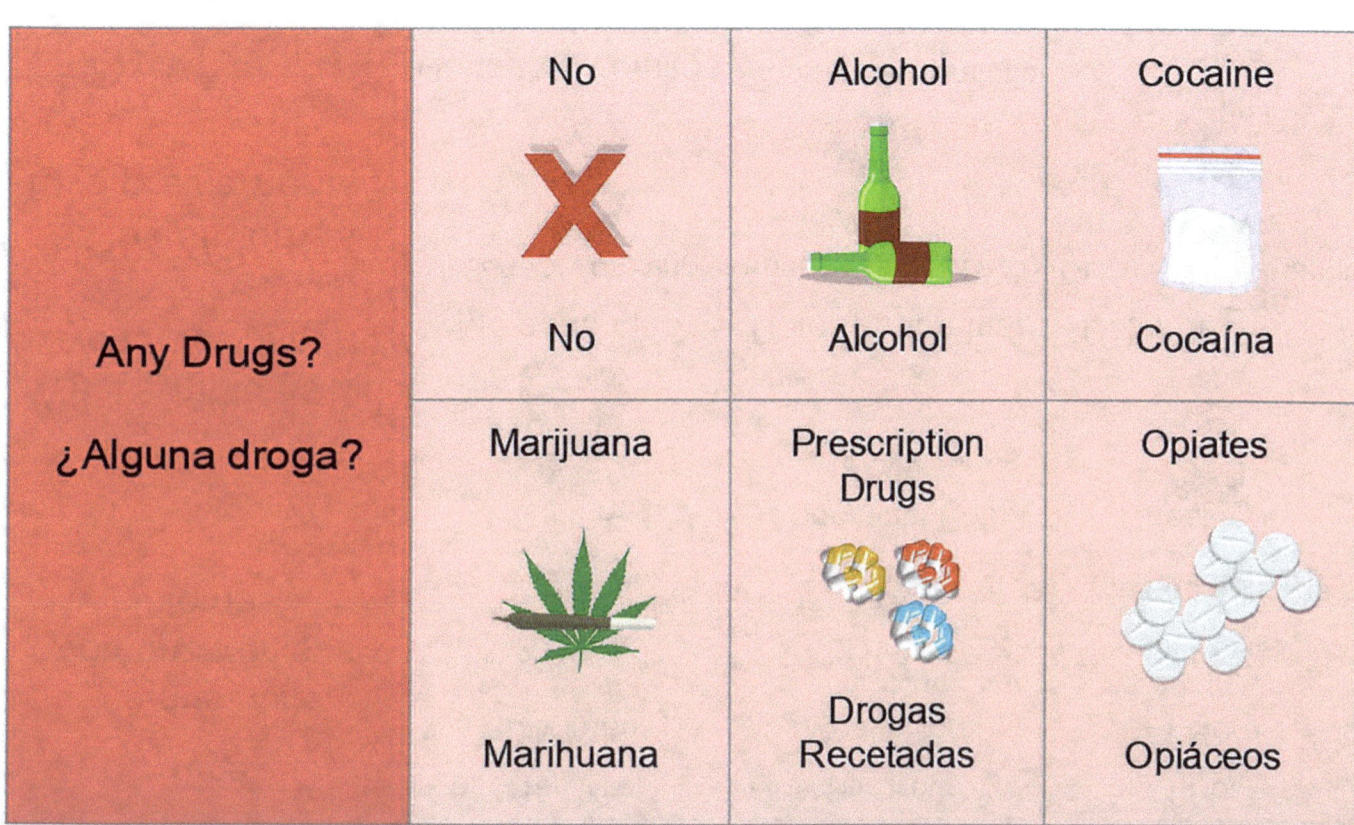

Any Drugs? ¿Alguna droga?	No X No	Alcohol Alcohol	Cocaine Cocaína
	Marijuana Marihuana	Prescription Drugs Drogas Recetadas	Opiates Opiáceos

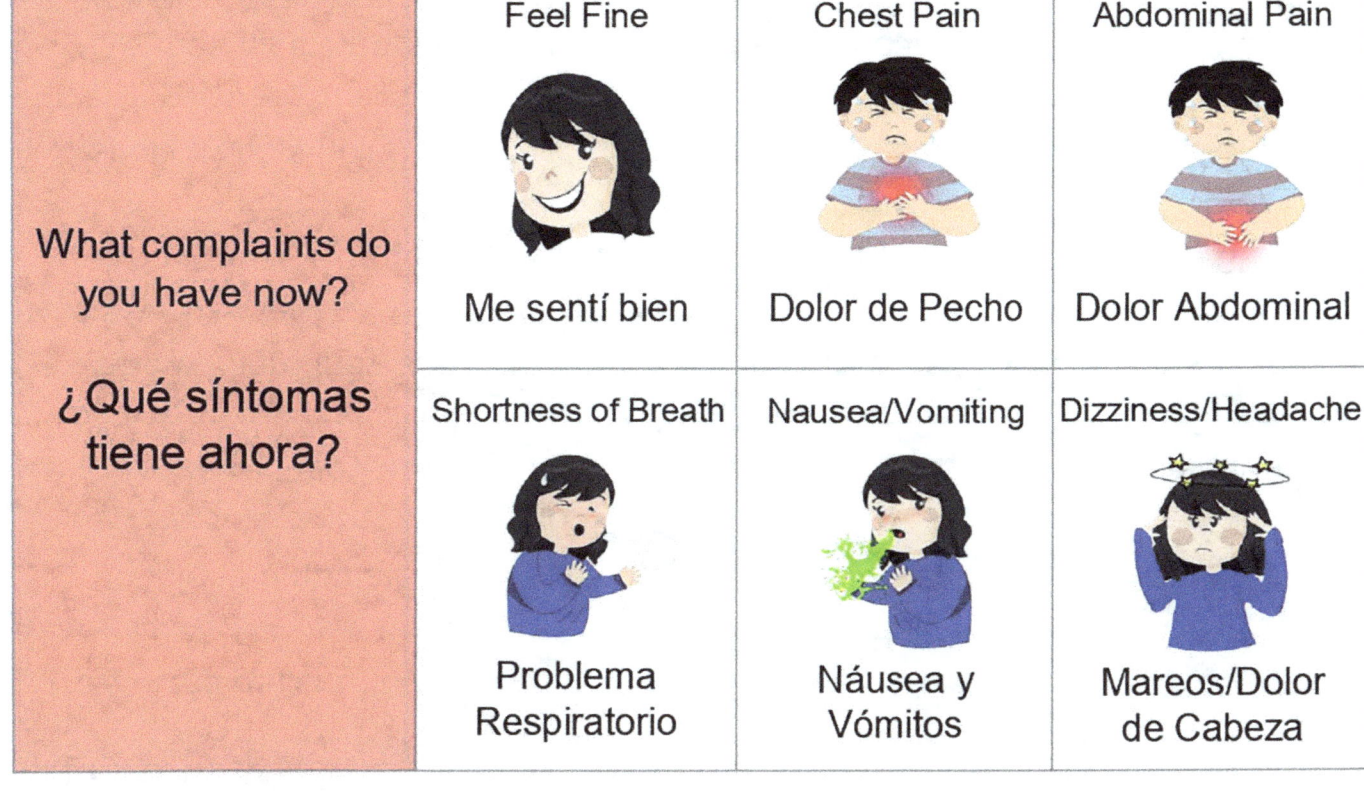

What complaints do you have now?

¿Qué síntomas tiene ahora?

Feel Fine	Chest Pain	Abdominal Pain
Me sentí bien	Dolor de Pecho	Dolor Abdominal
Shortness of Breath	Nausea/Vomiting	Dizziness/Headache
Problema Respiratorio	Náusea y Vómitos	Mareos/Dolor de Cabeza

ALOC/Stroke

How is the patient normally?	¿Cómo es el paciente normalmente?	Yes/Si No
Able to ambulate?	¿Puede caminar?	Yes/Si No
Know who they are?	¿Sabe quién es?	Yes/Si No
Know where they are?	¿Sabe quién es?	Yes/Si No
Know what year it is?	¿Sabe qué año es?	Yes/Si No
Know what is going on?	¿Sabe qué está sucediendo?	Yes/Si No
Did they hit their head?	¿Se golpeó la cabeza?	Yes/Si No

F	Can you smile for me?	¿Puede sonreír para mi?		
A	Can you stick both arms out and close your eyes?	¿Puede cerrar los ojos y poner ambos brazos rectos?		
S	Can you say: I like to eat spaghetti?	¿Puede decir?: Me gusta comer espagueti		
T	When were they last seen normal? ¿Cuándo fue la última vez que se lo/a vio normal?	10 Mins 10 Minutos	Half Hour Media Hora	1 Hour 1 Hora
		2-4 Hours 2-4 Horas	4-24 Hours 4-24 Horas	>24 Hours Más de 24 Horas

43

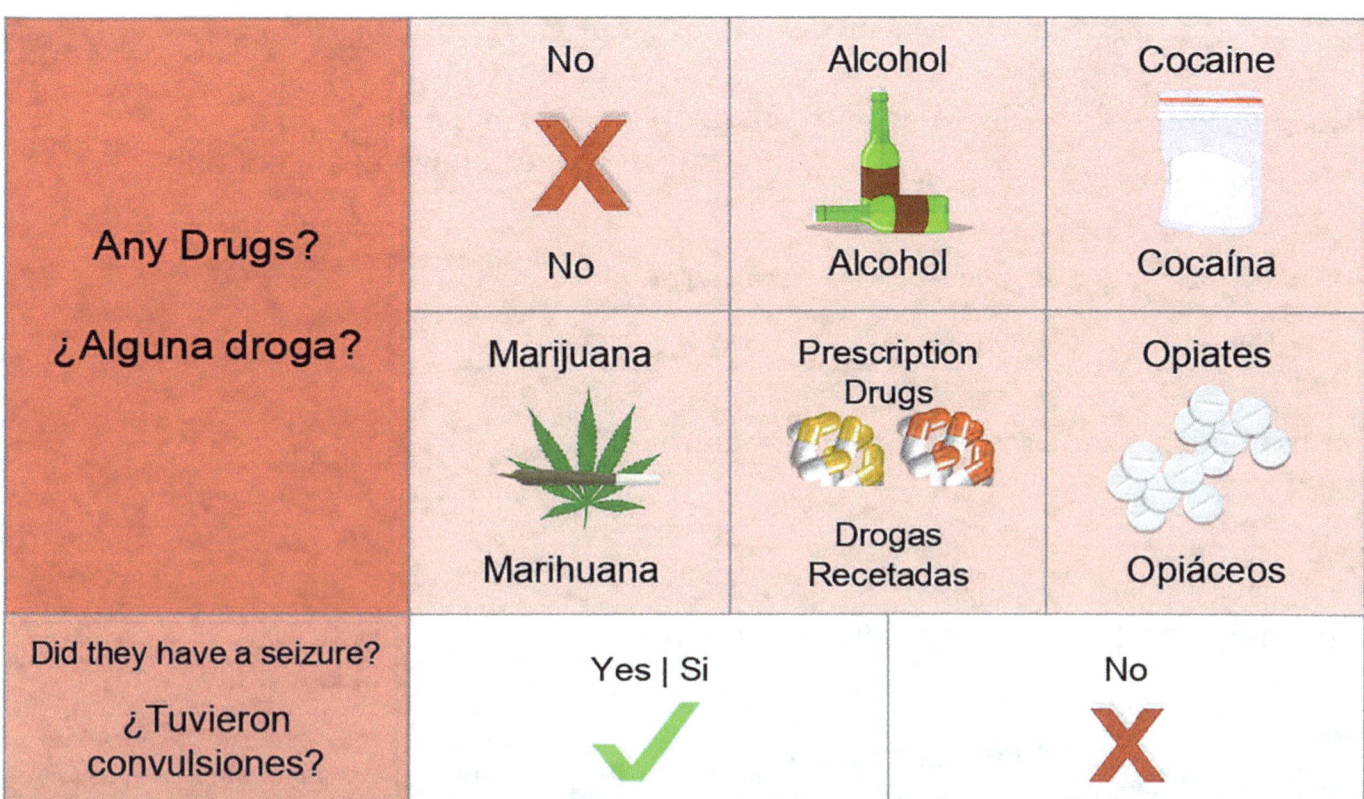

Any Drugs? ¿Alguna droga?	No **X** No	Alcohol Alcohol	Cocaine Cocaína
	Marijuana Marihuana	Prescription Drugs Drogas Recetadas	Opiates Opiáceos
Did they have a seizure? ¿Tuvieron convulsiones?	Yes | Si		No

44

Headache/Dizziness

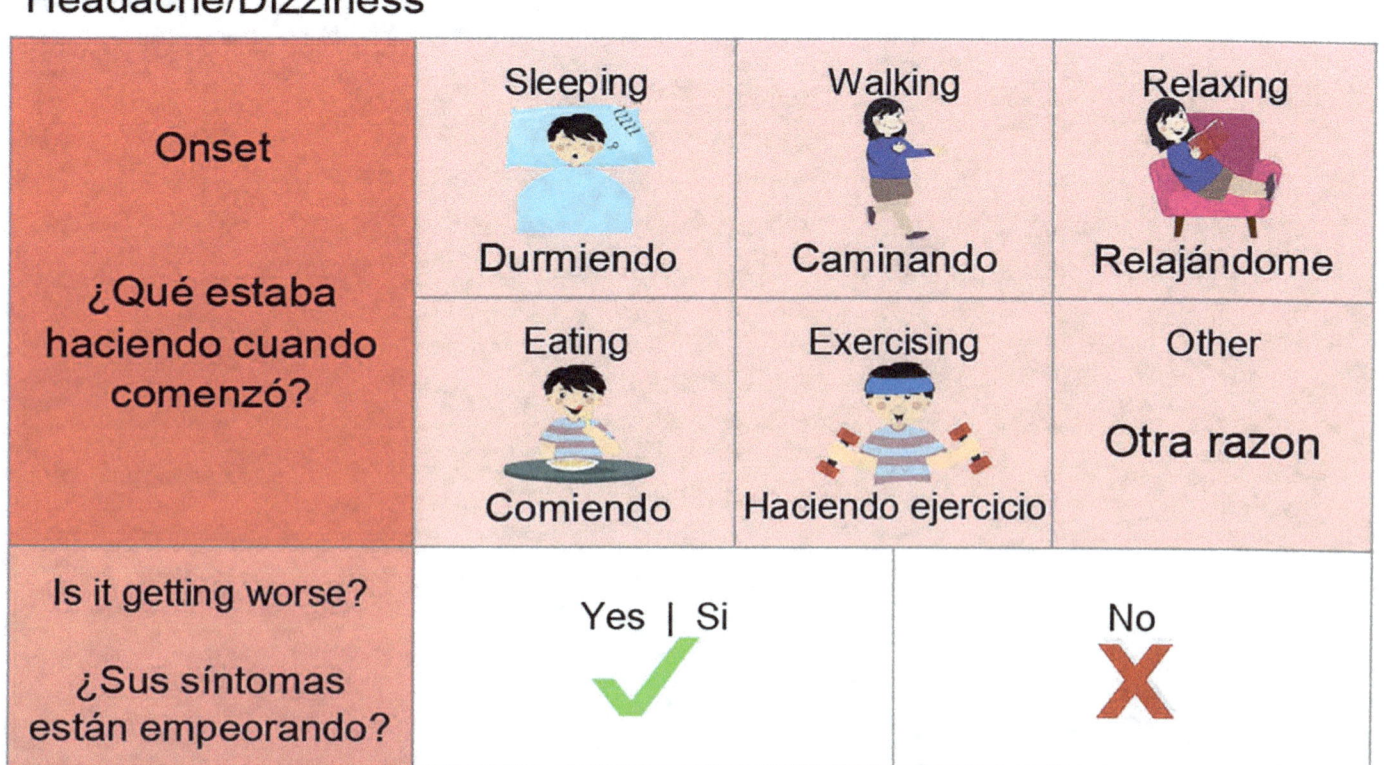

Onset ¿Qué estaba haciendo cuando comenzó?	Sleeping Durmiendo	Walking Caminando	Relaxing Relajándome
	Eating Comiendo	Exercising Haciendo ejercicio	Other Otra razon
Is it getting worse? ¿Sus síntomas están empeorando?	Yes | Si ✔		No ✗

Time ¿A qué hora comenzaron sus síntomas?	10 Mins 10 Minutos	Half Hour Media Hora	1 Hour 1 Hora
	2 Hours 2 Horas	3 Hours 3 Horas	>4 Hours Más de 4 Horas
Has this ever happened before? ¿Esto pasó antes alguna vez?	Yes | Si ✔️	No ✗	
Do you take your prescribed medications? ¿Toma sus medicamentos recetados?	Yes | Si ✔️	No ✗	

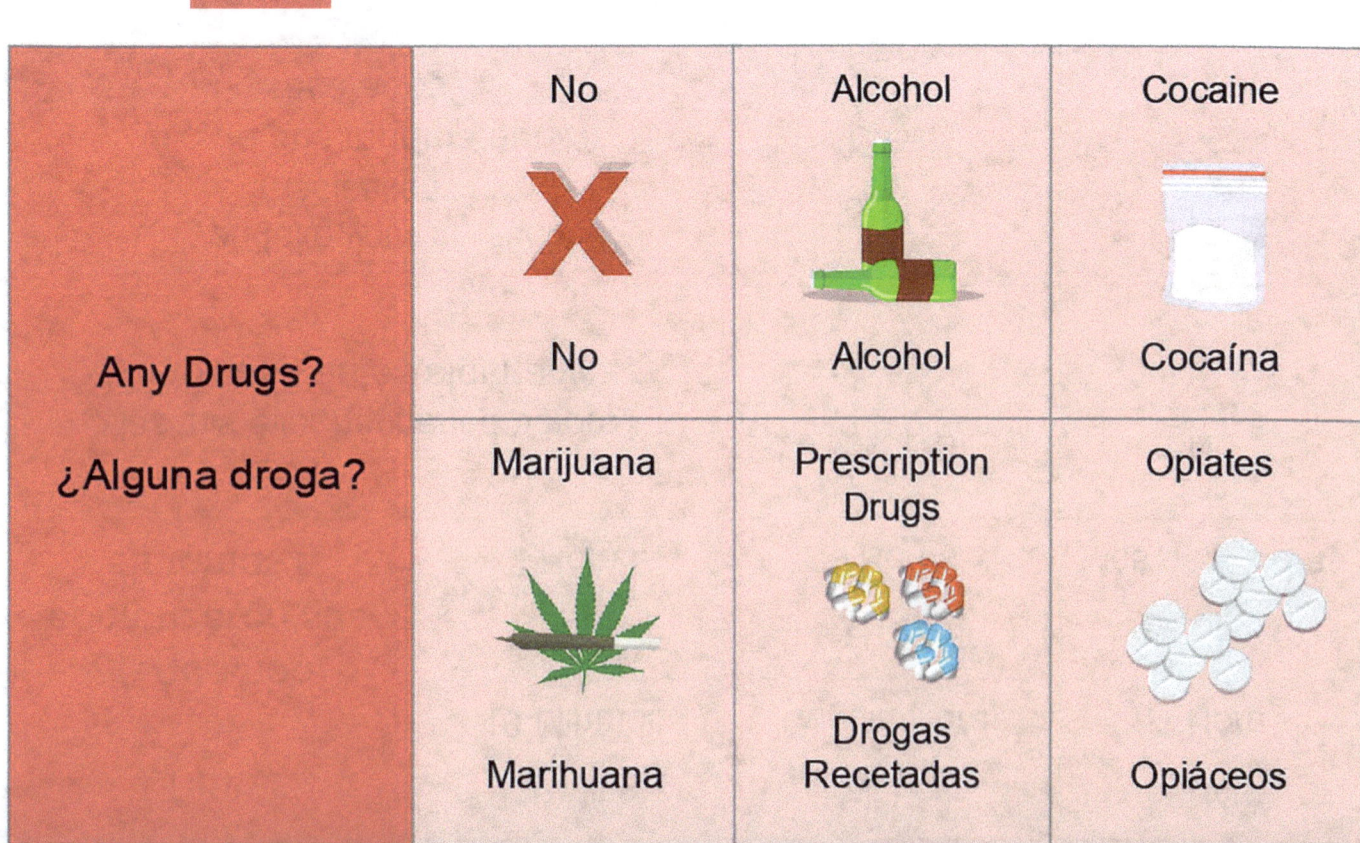

Any Drugs?

¿Alguna droga?

No / No

Alcohol / Alcohol

Cocaine / Cocaína

Marijuana / Marihuana

Prescription Drugs / Drogas Recetadas

Opiates / Opiáceos

Other complaints? ¿Algún Otro Síntoma?	Chest Pain Dolor de pecho	Abdominal Pain Dolor abdominal
No X	Shortness of Breath Problema respiratorio	Nausea/Vomiting Náusea y Vómitos
Other pain Otro Dolor	Syncope Desmayo	Headache/Dizziness Mareos/Dolor de Cabeza

46

Fall

Where are you hurting? ¿Dónde le duele?	No Injuries Sin lesiones		Can you point to where it hurts? ¿Puede señalar dónde le duele?	
When did it happen? ¿Cuando esto pasó?	10 Mins 10 Minutos	Half Hour Media Hora	1 Hour 1 Hora	
	2 Hours 2 Horas	3 Hours 3 Horas	>4 Hours Mas de 4 Horas	
Did you lose consciousness? ¿Perdió el conocimiento?	Yes | Si For how long? ¿Por cuánto tiempo perdió el conocimiento?		No Are they behaving normal now? ¿Se está comportando de modo normal ahora?	

Height of Fall?	1 Feet 1 Pie	2-3 Feet 2-3 Pies	4-5 Feet 4-5 Pies
¿Altura de caída?	6-10 Feet 6-10 Pies	11-15 Feet 11-15 Pies	>20 Feet 20 Pies
Why did you fall?	Trip & Fall/Rolled out of Bed Tropezón y caída/Bajando de la cama		Weakness/Dizziness Debilidad/Mareos
¿Por qué se cayó?	Fainting/Syncope Desmayo/Síncope		Other Reason Otra razón
Are you on any blood thinning medications? ¿Toma alguna medicación anticoagulante?	Yes/Si Can we see the medications? ¿Podemos ver sus medicamentos?		No. Can we see the medications? No. ¿Podemos ver sus medicamentos?

47

Trauma

What happened? ¿Qué sucedió?	Assault Ataque	Motor-vehicle Accident Accidente de Vehículo a Motor
	Motor-vehicle vs Person Accidente de Vehículo a Motor vs. Peatón	Other Reason Otra Razón

Where are you hurting? ¿Dónde le duele?	No Injuries Sin lesiones		Can you point to where it hurts? ¿Puede señalar dónde le duele?	
When did it happen? ¿Cuando esto pasó?	10 Mins 10 Minutos	Half Hour Media Hora	1 Hour 1 Hora	
	2 Hours 2 Horas	3 Hours 3 Horas	>4 Hours Más de 4 Horas	
Did you lose consciousness? ¿Perdió el conocimiento?	Yes | Si ✅		No ❌	

48

Were you wearing your seatbelt? ¿Llevaba puesto el cinturón de seguridad?	Yes | Si ✔		No ✗	
Speed of Vehicle Velocidad del Vehículo	5-10 MPH 5-10 millas por hora	10-15 MPH 10-15 millas por hora	15-20 MPH 15-20 millas por hora	
	20-30 MPH 20-30 millas por hora	30-40 MPH 30-40 millas por hora	Above 50 MPH Más de 50 millas por hora	

Are you on any blood thinning medications? ¿Toma alguna medicación anticoagulante?	Yes | Si Can we see the medications? ¿Podemos ver sus medicamentos?	No Can we see the medications? ¿Podemos ver sus medicamentos?

Miscellaneous Questions

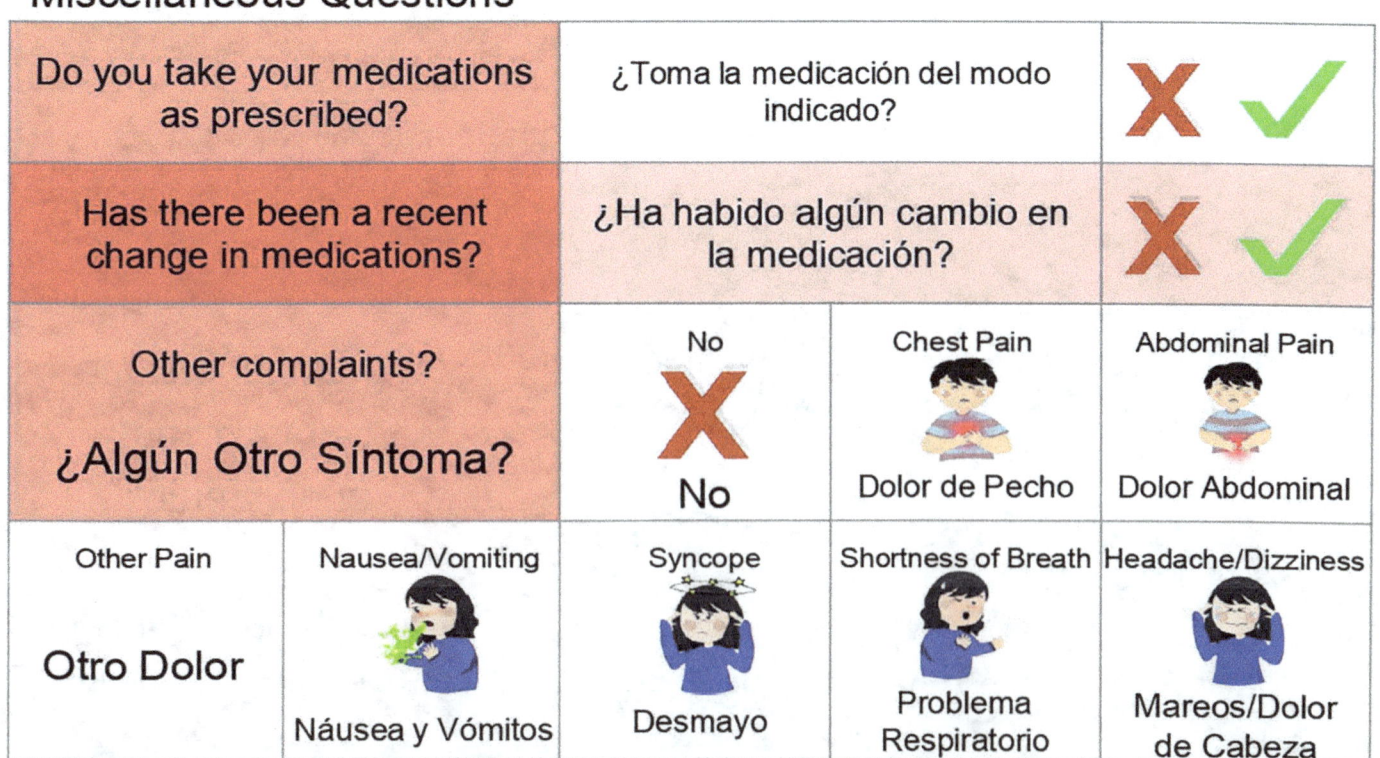

Do you take your medications as prescribed?	¿Toma la medicación del modo indicado?	✗ ✓	
Has there been a recent change in medications?	¿Ha habido algún cambio en la medicación?	✗ ✓	
Other complaints? ¿Algún Otro Síntoma?	No ✗ No	Chest Pain Dolor de Pecho	Abdominal Pain Dolor Abdominal
Other Pain Otro Dolor	Nausea/Vomiting Náusea y Vómitos	Syncope Desmayo	Shortness of Breath Problema Respiratorio
			Headache/Dizziness Mareos/Dolor de Cabeza

When was the last time you ate something? ¿Cuándo fue la última vez que comió algo?	10 Mins 10 Minutos	Half Hour Media Hora	1 Hour 1 Hora
	2 Hours 2 Horas	3 Hours 3 Horas	>4 Hours Más de 4 Horas
Have you ever felt this way before?	¿Alguna vez se sintió así antes?		X ✔
Does the patient have a DNR order?	¿Tiene el paciente una Orden de No Resucitar?		X ✔
Do you want to go to the hospital?	¿Quiere ir al hospital?		X ✔

50

Medical History - Historia clínica. Elija lo que tiene de la listatiene.

Asthma	Asma
Atrial Fibrillation	Fibrilación Auricular
Cancer	Cáncer
COPD	EPOC
Diabetes	Diabetes
Hypertension	Hipertensión
Heart Failure	Falla Cardíaca

Liver Problems	Problemas de Hígado
Myocardial Infarctions	Ataques Cardíacos Previos
Renal Problems	Problemas Renales
Seizures	Convulsiones
Stroke	Ataque Cerebral

51

Medications - Medicamentos. Elija lo que toma de la lista

Aspirin	Aspirina
Atorvastatin	Atorvastatina
Benadryl	Benadryl
Blood Thinners	Anticoagulantes
Erythromycin	Eritromicina
Fentanyl	Fentanilo
Insulin	Insulin

Ketamine	Ketamina
Metformin	Metformina
Metoprolol	Metoprolol
Morphine	Morfina
Penicillin	Penicilina
Sulfa Drugs	Sulfamida
Warfarin	Warfarina

52

Allergies - Alergias. Elija lo que toma de la lista

No Known Drug Allergies	Sin alergias a medicamentos
Aspirin	Aspirina
Atorvastatin	Atorvastatina
Benadryl	Benadryl
Blood Thinners	Anticoagulantes
Erythromycin	Eritromicina
Fentanyl	Fentanilo

Ketamine	Ketamina
Metformin	Metformina
Metoprolol	Metoprolol
Morphine	Morfina
Penicillin	Penicilina
Sulfa Drugs	Sulfamida
Warfarin	Warfarina

53

Intervention Phrases

I am going to start a IV on you	Voy a colocarle una vía endovenosa
I am going to check your blood sugar	Voy a revisar su nivel de azúcar
I am going to put a collar around your neck	Voy a colocarle un collar cervical alrededor del cuello
I am going to assess your heart, these stickers are going to be on your left chest	Voy a evaluar su corazón, estas pegatinas van a ir en su pecho izquierdo

I am going to give you a medication. Let me know if your symptoms get better or worst	Voy a darle una medicación. Cuénteme si sus síntomas mejoran o empeoran
How are you feeling now? ¿Cómo se siente ahora?	0 2 4 6 8 10

54

Russian

Русский

Hello I am a medical professional. I do not speak your language, but I will be using this translation guide to help me. Please read the question and point to the correct choice

Здравствуйте, я медицинский работник. Я не знаю вашего языка. Для общения с вами я буду пользоваться этим руководством. Пожалуйста, прочтите вопрос и выберите один из предложенных вариантов

Alert & Oriented Questions

What is your name?	Как вас зовут?	
Where are we now? **Где мы находимся?**	House Дом	Restaurant Ресторан	Outside На улице
	Store Магазин	Ambulance Больница	Other Другое место

What time of day is it? Какое сейчас время суток?	Morning Утро	Afternoon День	Evening Вечер
Who are we? Знаете, кто я?	Mom Мать	Chef Повар	Farmer Фермер
	Paramedic Врач	Dad Отец	Construction Worker Строитель

Chief Complaints

What's going on today?	На что вы жалуетесь?
Chest Pain | p. 58-59 Боль в груди	Abdominal Pain | p. 60-61 Боль в животе
Other Pains | p. 62-63 Другие боли	Breathing Difficulty | p.64-65 Проблемы с дыханием

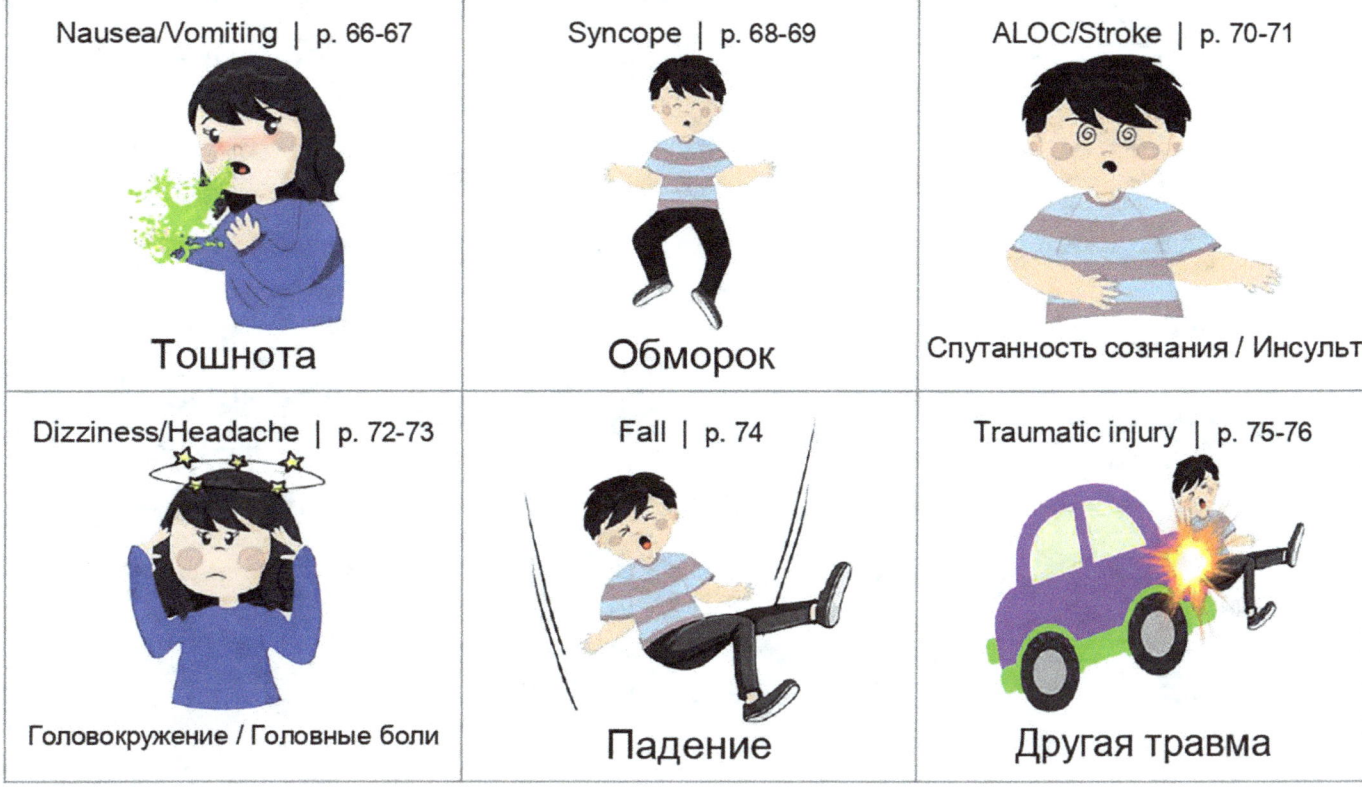

Nausea/Vomiting | p. 66-67

Тошнота

Syncope | p. 68-69

Обморок

ALOC/Stroke | p. 70-71

Спутанность сознания / Инсульт

Dizziness/Headache | p. 72-73

Головокружение / Головные боли

Fall | p. 74

Падение

Traumatic injury | p. 75-76

Другая травма

Chest Pain

Onset Чем вы занимались, когда появилась боль?	Sleeping Сон	Walking Прогулка	Relaxing Отдых
	Eating Еда	Exercising Физическая нагрузка	Other Другое

How did it develop? Как возникла боль?	Gradual Постепенно	Sudden Внезапно

Provocation Что усиливает боль?	Movement Движение	Breathing Дыхание	Pressure Давление	Constant Постоянная боль
Quality Какой у вас тип боли?	Palpitations Учащенное сердцебиение	Sharp Острая боль	Crushing Давящая боль	
	Dull Ноющая боль	Burning Жгучая боль	Stabbing Колющая боль	

Chest Pain (continued)

Radiation: Point to where it hurts most and where the pain travels to	Пожалуйста, покажите, что больше всего болит и куда боль переходит				
Severity ? Как сильно ощущается боль?	0	2	4	6	8	10

Time В какое время начали проявляться симптомы?	10 Mins 10 минут	Half Hour Полчаса	1 Hour 1 час
	2 Hours 2 часа	3 Hours 3 часа	>4 Hours 4 часа

Pertinent Negatives: Are you having any of the following Есть ли у вас следующие симптомы?	Нет X	Abdominal Pain Боль в животе	Breathing Difficulty Проблемы с дыханием
		Nausea/Vomiting Тошнота и рвота	Other Pains Другие боли

Abdominal Pain

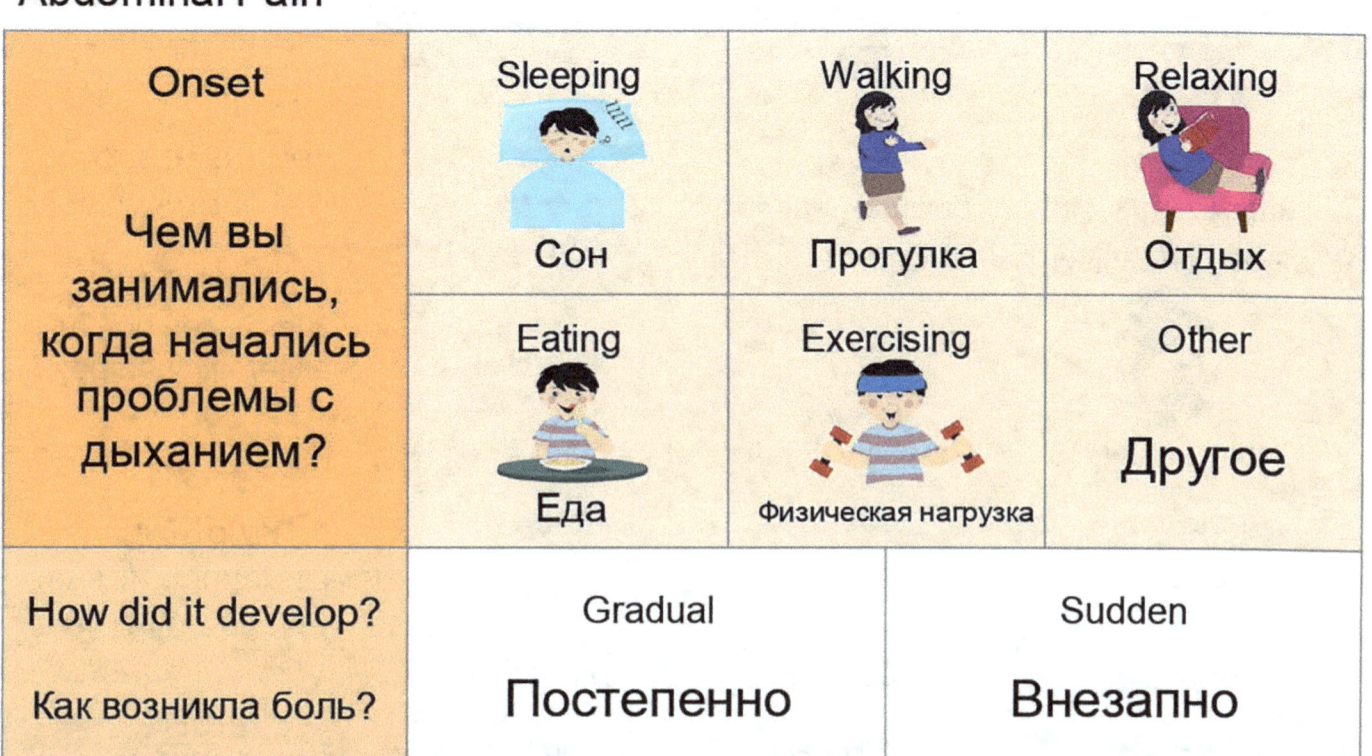

Onset Чем вы занимались, когда начались проблемы с дыханием?	Sleeping Сон	Walking Прогулка	Relaxing Отдых
	Eating Еда	Exercising Физическая нагрузка	Other Другое
How did it develop? Как возникла боль?	Gradual Постепенно		Sudden Внезапно

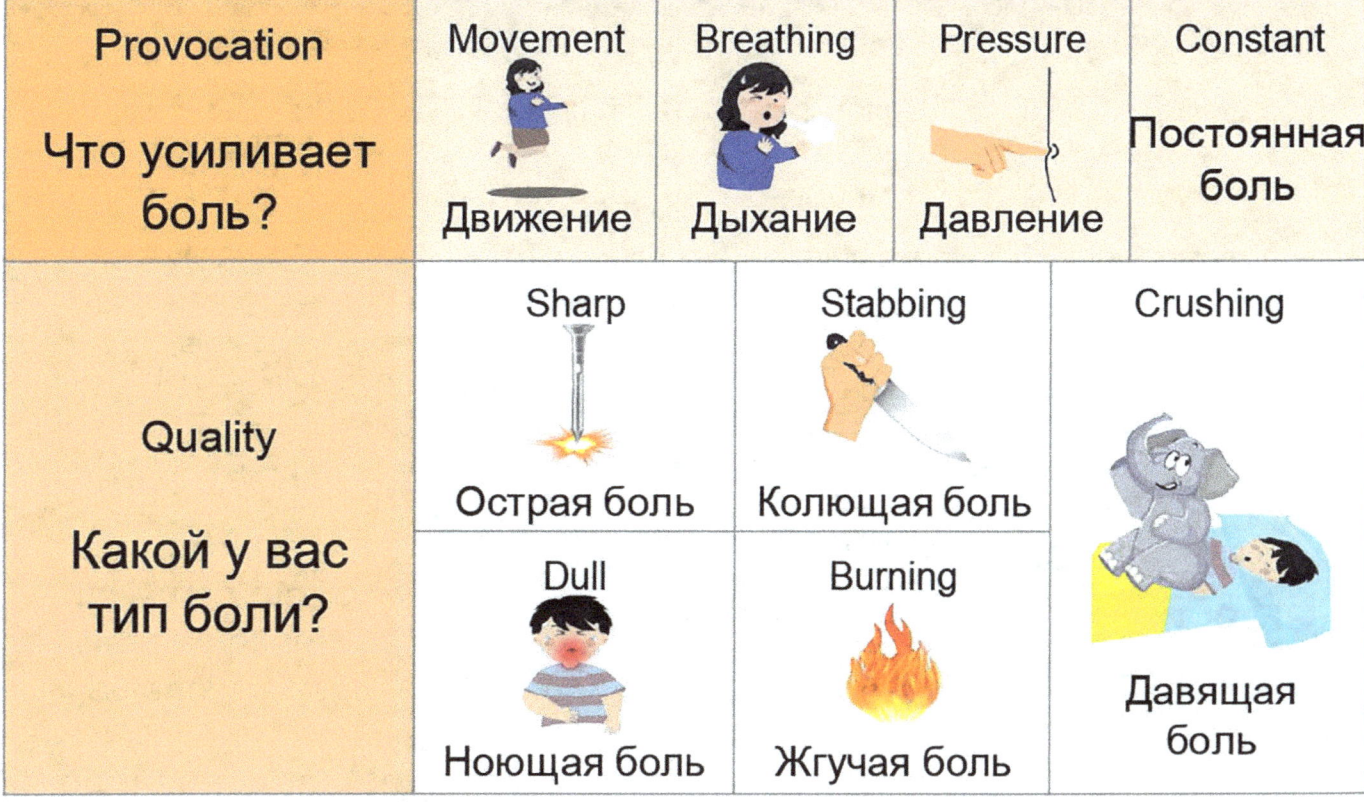

Provocation Что усиливает боль?	Movement Движение	Breathing Дыхание	Pressure Давление	Constant Постоянная боль
Quality Какой у вас тип боли?	Sharp Острая боль	Stabbing Колющая боль	Crushing Давящая боль	
	Dull Ноющая боль	Burning Жгучая боль		

Abdominal Pain (continued)

Radiation: Point to where it hurts most and where the pain travels to	Покажите, в какой части тела боль ощущается больше всего и куда она переходит					
Severity ? Как сильно ощущается боль?	0 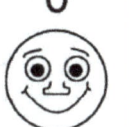	2 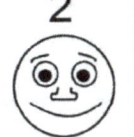	4 	6 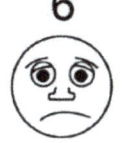	8 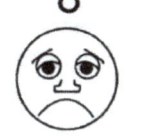	10 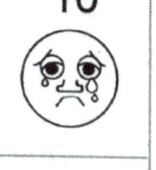
Time Как давно начали проявляться симптомы?	10 Mins 10 минут	Half Hour Полчаса		1 Hour 1 час		
	2 Hours 2 часа	3 Hours 3 часа		>4 Hours Более 4 часов		

Is there any chance you are pregnant? Есть ли вероятность, что вы беременны?	Yes | Да ✓	No I Нет X
Pertinent Negatives/ Are you having any of the following? **Есть ли у вас следующие симптомы?**	Нет 	**Abdominal Pain** 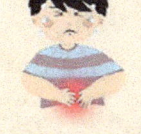 Боль в животе	**Breathing Difficulty** 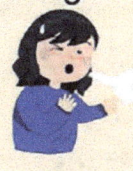 Проблемы с дыханием
	Nausea/Vomiting 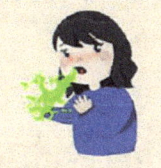 Тошнота и рвота	Diarrhea/Constipation 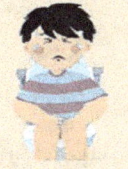 Диарея/запор	Other Pains 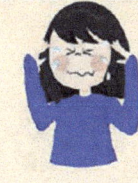 Другие боли

Other Pains

Onset Что вы делали, когда началась боль?	Sleeping Сон	Walking Прогулка	Relaxing Отдых
	Eating Еда	Exercising Физическая нагрузка	Other Другое
How did it develop? Как начиналась боль?	Gradual Постепенно	Sudden Внезапно	

Provocation Чем вы занимались, когда появилась боль?	Movement 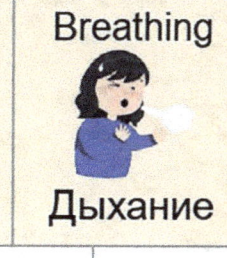 Движение	Breathing 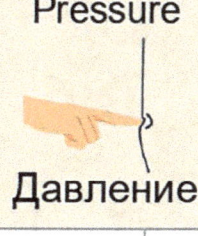 Дыхание	Pressure 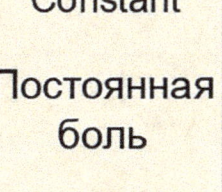 Давление	Constant Постоянная боль
Quality **Какой у вас тип боли?**	Sharp Острая боль Dull Ноющая боль	Stabbing Колющая боль Burning Жгучая боль	Crushing Давящая боль	

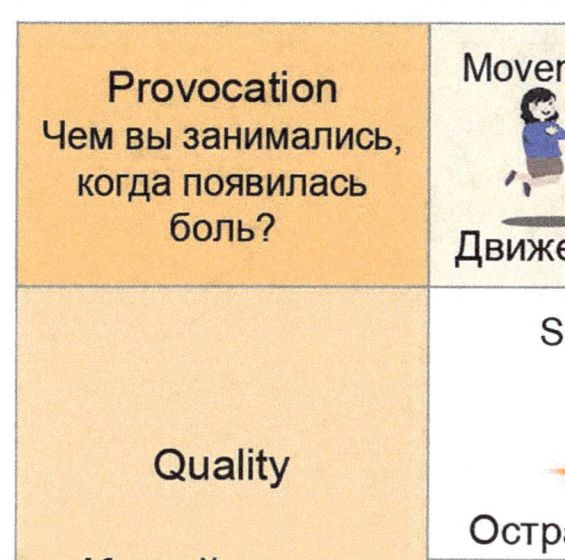
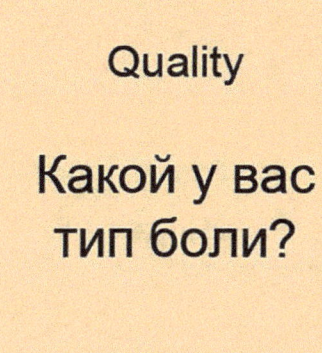
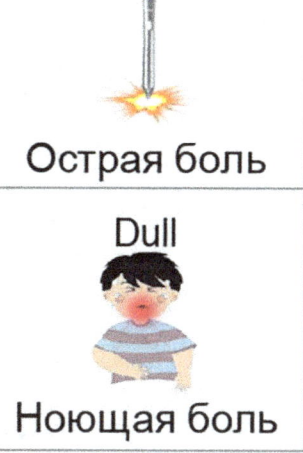

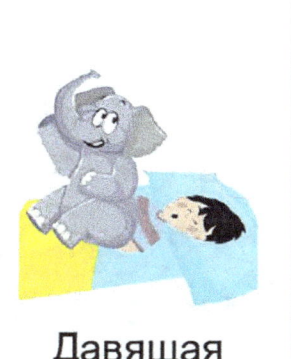

Other Pains (continued)

Radiation: Point to where it hurts most and where the pain travels to	Покажите, в какой части тела боль ощущается больше всего и куда она переходит				
Severity ? **Как сильно ощущаетс я боль?**	0	2	4	6	8	10

Time Как давно начали проявляться симптомы?	10 Mins 10 минут	Half Hour Полчаса	1 Hour 1 час
	2 Hours 2 часа	3 Hours 3 часа	>4 Hours Более 4 часов
Pertinent Negatives/ Are you having any of the following? Есть ли у вас следующие симптомы?	No X Нет	Abdominal Pain Боль в животе	Breathing Difficulty Проблемы с дыханием
	Nausea/Vomiting Тошнота и рвота	Diarrhea/Constipation Диарея/запор	Other Pains Другие боли

Shortness of Breath

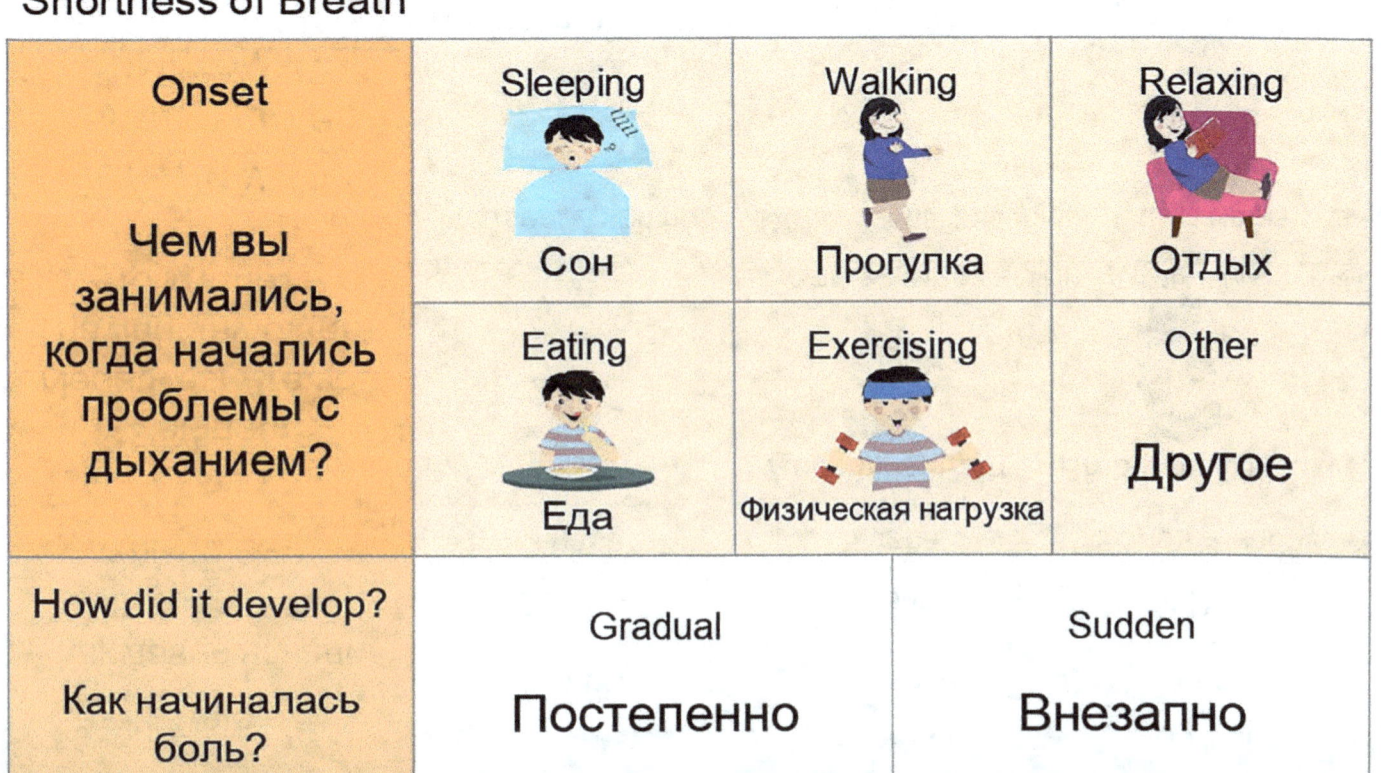

Onset Чем вы занимались, когда начались проблемы с дыханием?	Sleeping Сон	Walking Прогулка	Relaxing Отдых
	Eating Еда	Exercising Физическая нагрузка	Other Другое
How did it develop? Как начиналась боль?	Gradual Постепенно		Sudden Внезапно

Do you have associated chest pain? Ощущаете ли вы боль в груди?	Yes | Да ✔	No | Нет ✗

Sputum: Are you coughing, what color is your phlegm? Вы кашляете? Какого цвета мокрота при кашле?	None ✗ Нет	Dry Cough 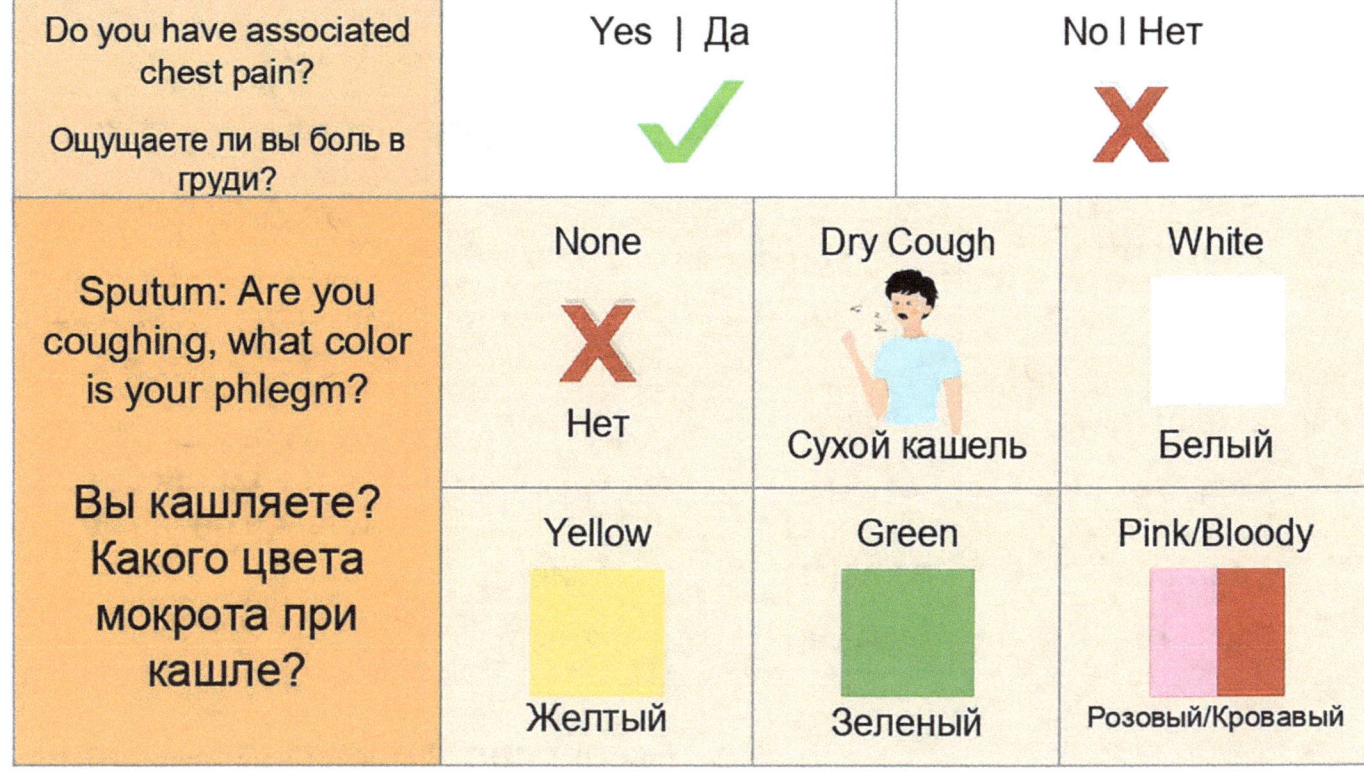 Сухой кашель	White ⬜ Белый
	Yellow 🟨 Желтый	Green 🟩 Зеленый	Pink/Bloody 🟪🟥 Розовый/Кровавый

Shortness of Breath (continued)

Time Как давно начали проявляться симптомы?	10 Mins 10 минут	Half Hour Полчаса	1 Hour 1 час
	2 Hours 2 часа	3 Hours 3 часа	>4 Hours Более 4 часов
Exertion: Does movement and exercise make it worse? При движении и физических нагрузках усиливаются проблемы с дыханием?	Yes | Да ✔	No | Нет ✘	

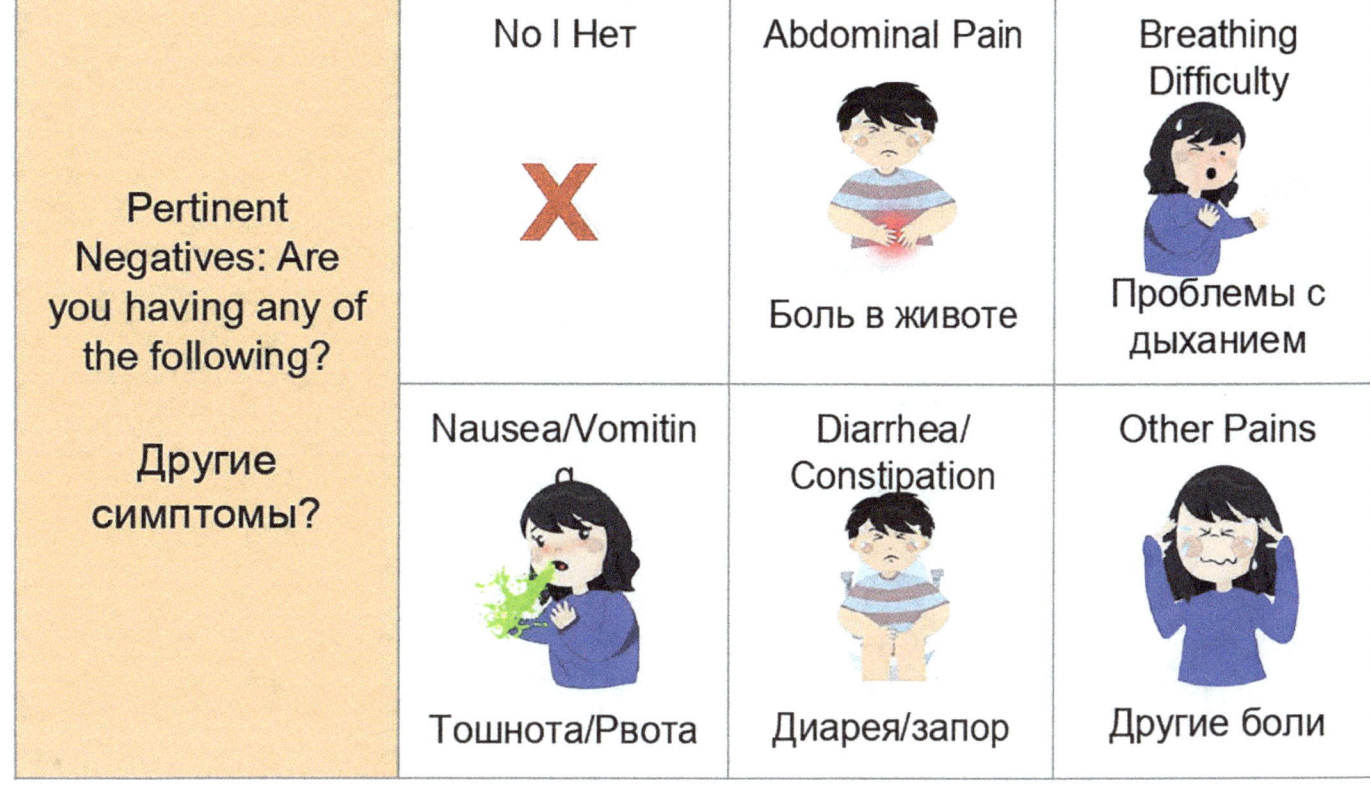

Pertinent Negatives: Are you having any of the following? Другие симптомы?	No I Нет X	Abdominal Pain Боль в животе	Breathing Difficulty Проблемы с дыханием
	Nausea/Vomiting Тошнота/Рвота	Diarrhea/ Constipation Диарея/запор	Other Pains Другие боли

Nausea and Vomiting

Onset Чем вы занимались, когда начались проблемы с дыханием?	Sleeping 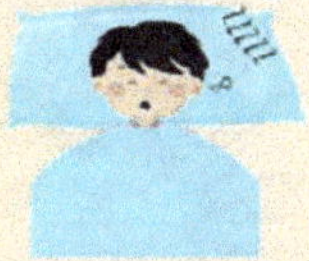 Сон	Walking 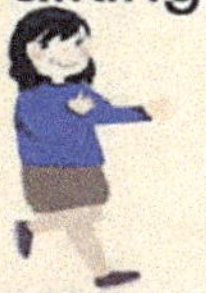 Прогулка	Relaxing 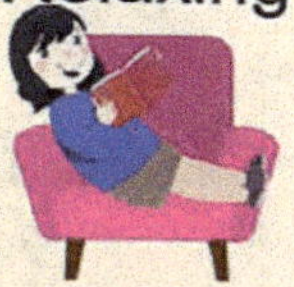 Отдых
	Eating 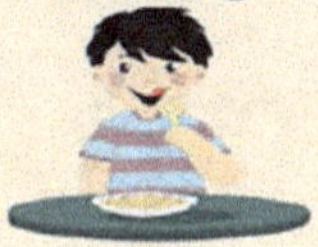 Еда	Exercising 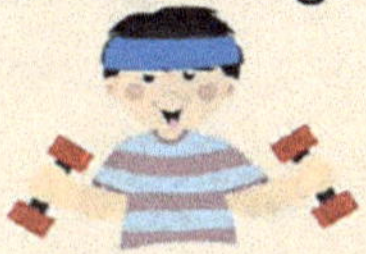 Физическая нагрузка	Other Другое
Is there any blood in your vomit? Есть ли кровь в рвоте?	Yes | Да ✅		No I Нет 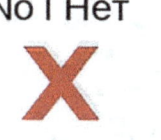

Time Как давно начали проявляться симптомы?	10 Mins 10 минут	Half Hour Полчаса	1 Hour 1 час
	2 Hours 2 часа	3 Hours 3 часа	>4 Hours Более 4 часов

Are you having abdominal pain? Ощущаете ли вы боль в животе?	Yes | Да ✅		No I Нет ❌

Are you pregnant? Есть ли вероятность, что вы беременны?	Yes | Да ✅ How many months? На каком вы месяце беременности?		No I Нет ❌

Nausea and Vomiting (Continued)

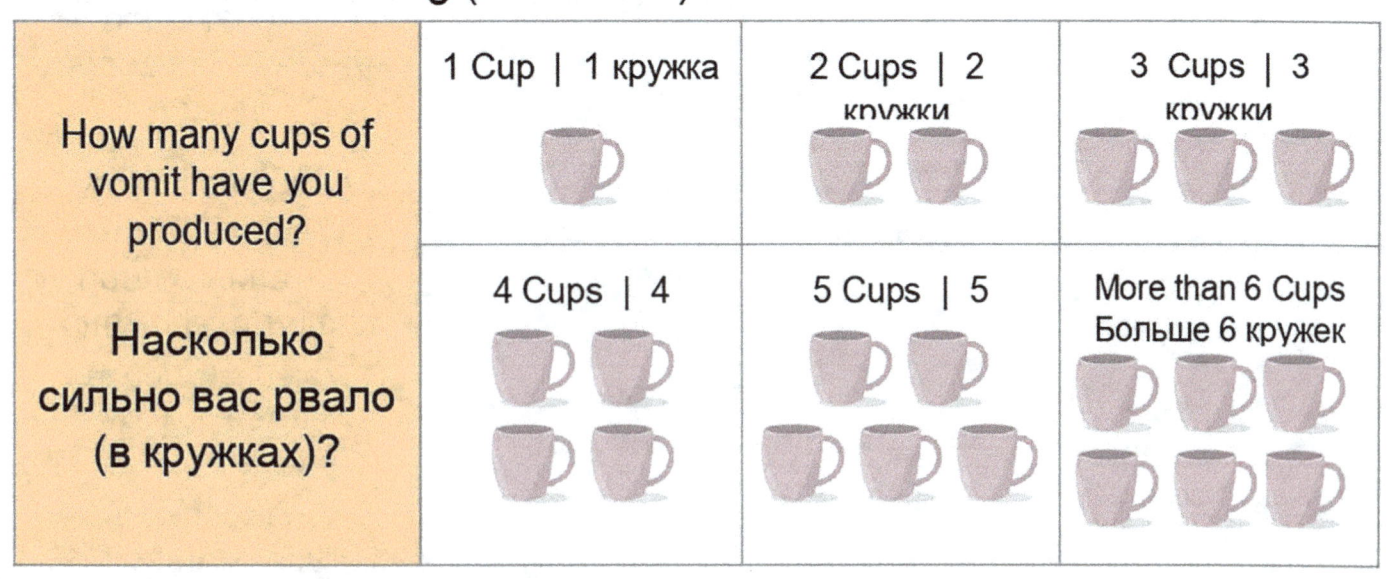

How many cups of vomit have you produced? Насколько сильно вас рвало (в кружках)?	1 Cup | 1 кружка	2 Cups | 2 кружки	3 Cups | 3 кружки
	4 Cups | 4	5 Cups | 5	More than 6 Cups Больше 6 кружек

	No I Нет	Abdominal Pain	Breathing Difficulty
Pertinent Negatives: Are you having any of the following? **Есть ли у вас следующие симптомы?**	**X**	Боль в животе	Проблемы с дыханием
	Nausea/Vomitin Тошнота и рвота	Diarrhea/ Constipation Диарея/запор	Other Pains Другие боли

Syncope

Onset	Sleeping	Walking	Relaxing
Чем вы занимались, когда начались проблемы с дыханием?	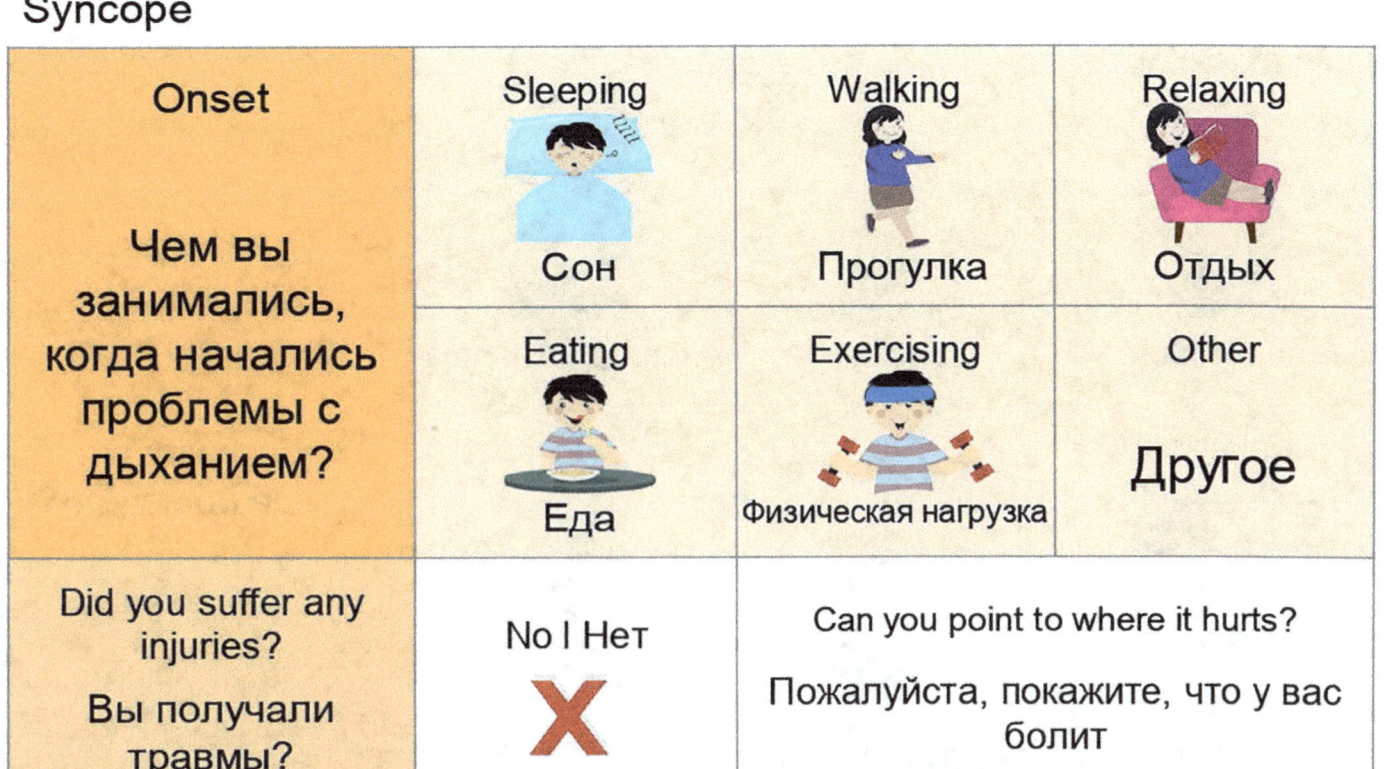 Сон	Прогулка	Отдых
	Eating Еда	Exercising Физическая нагрузка	Other Другое
Did you suffer any injuries? Вы получали травмы?	No I Нет X	Can you point to where it hurts? Пожалуйста, покажите, что у вас болит	

Time Как давно начали проявляться симптомы?	10 Mins 10 минут	Half Hour Полчаса	1 Hour 1 час
	2 Hours 2 часа	3 Hours 3 часа	>4 Hours Более 4 часов

What symptoms did you have prior? Какие симптомы у вас были до этого?	Felt Fine Все было хорошо	Abdominal Pain Боль в животе	Chest Pain Боль в груди
	Nausea/Vomiting Тошнота и рвота	Shortness of Breath Проблемы с дыханием	Dizziness/Headache Головокружение / Головные боли

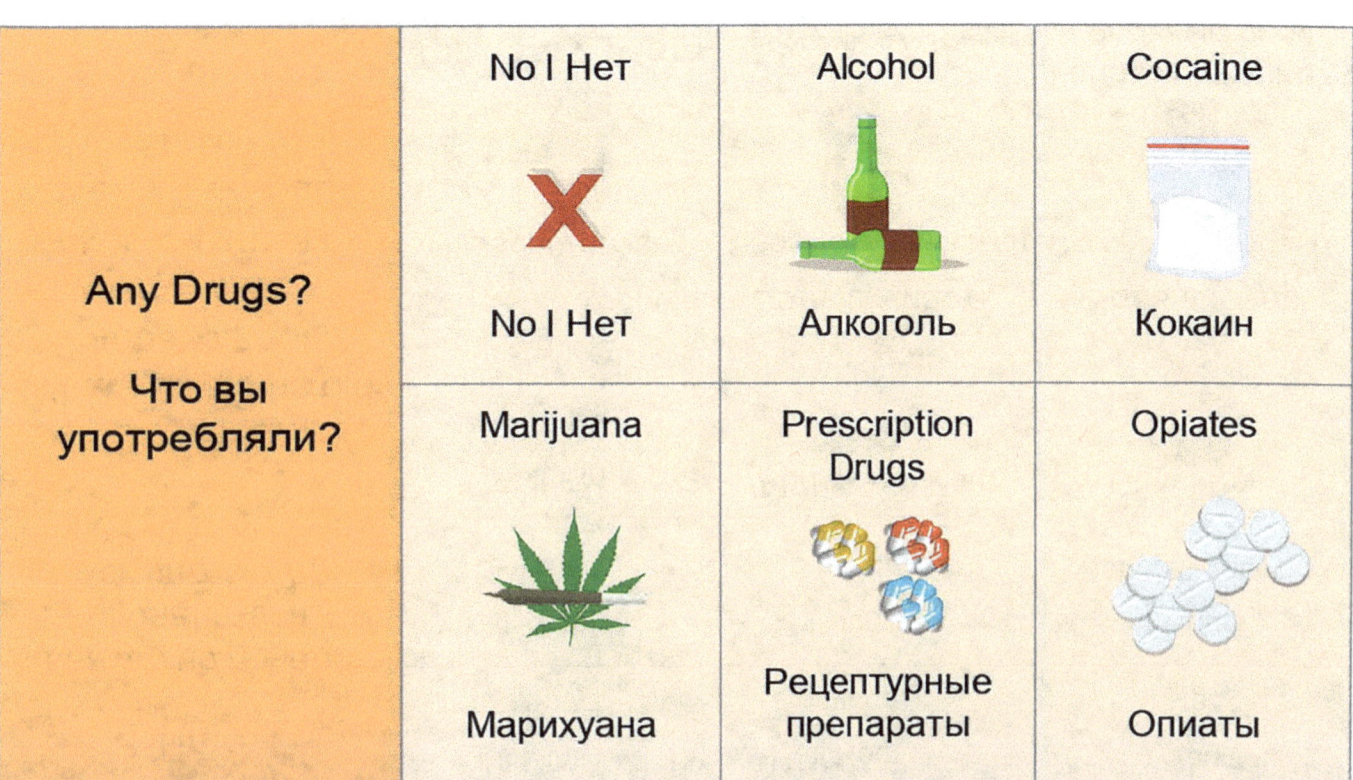

Any Drugs? Что вы употребляли?	No l Нет **X** No l Нет	Alcohol Алкоголь	Cocaine Кокаин
	Marijuana Марихуана	Prescription Drugs Рецептурные препараты	Opiates Опиаты

What complaints do you have now? Какие симптомы у вас сейчас?	Feel Fine 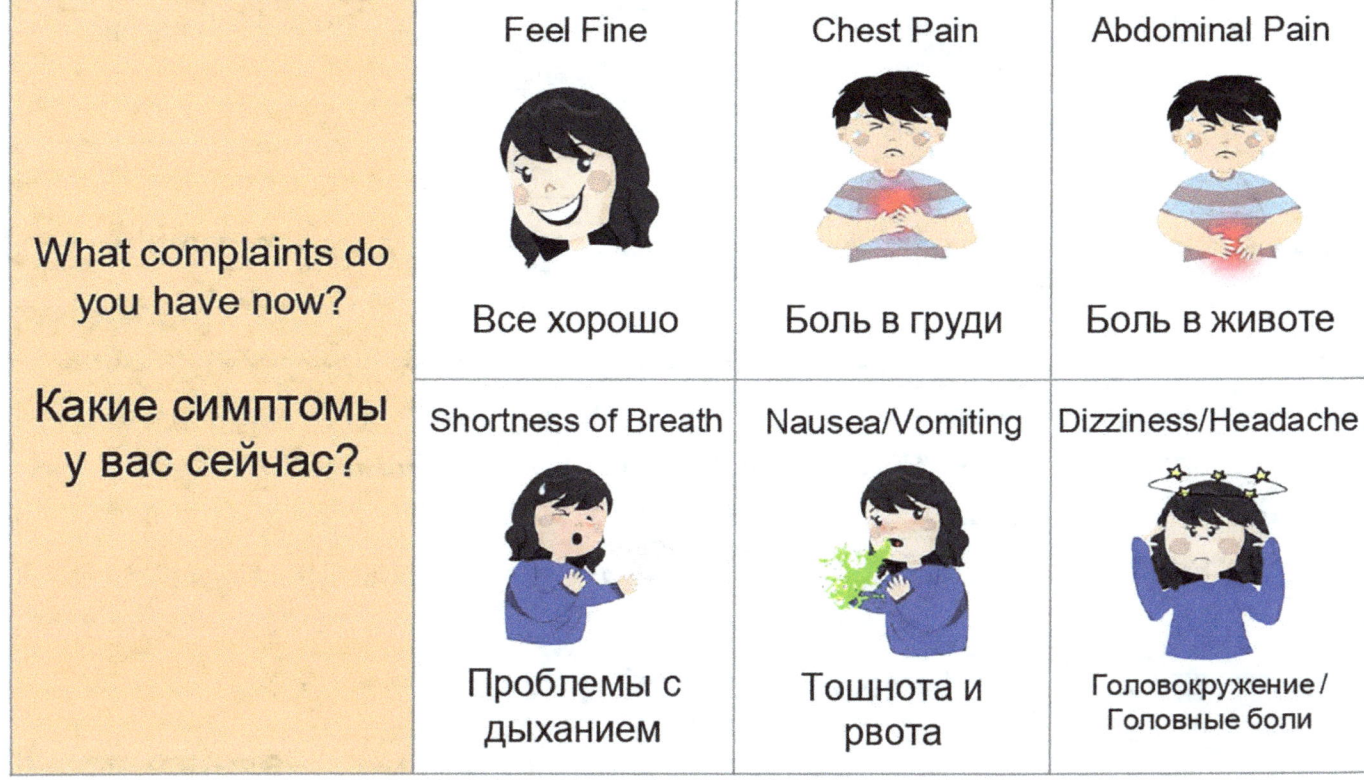 Все хорошо	Chest Pain Боль в груди	Abdominal Pain Боль в животе
	Shortness of Breath Проблемы с дыханием	Nausea/Vomiting Тошнота и рвота	Dizziness/Headache Головокружение / Головные боли

ALOC/Stroke

How is the patient normally?	Как обычно ведет себя пациент?	Yes/Да No/ Нет
Able to ambulate?	Способен ли он передвигаться?	Yes/Да No/ Нет
Know who they are?	Понимает, кто он/она?	Yes/Да No/ Нет
Know where they are?	Понимает, где он/она?	Yes/Да No/ Нет
Know what year it is?	Знает, какой сейчас год?	Yes/Да No/ Нет
Know what is going on?	Понимает, что происходит?	Yes/Да No/ Нет
Did they hit their head?	Получал(-а) ли он/она травму головы?	Yes/Да No/ Нет

F	Can you smile for me?	Не могли бы вы улыбнуться?
A	Can you stick both arms out and close your eyes?	Не могли бы вы закрыть глаза и вытянуть руки?
S	Can you say: I like to eat spaghetti?	Пожалуйста, скажите: «Я люблю макароны»

		10 Mins 10 минут	Half Hour Полчаса	1 Hour 1 час
T	When were they last seen normal? Когда он/она чувствовал(-а) себя нормально в последний раз?	2-4 Hours 2-4 часа	4-24 Hours 4-24 часа	>24 Hours Более 24 часов

70

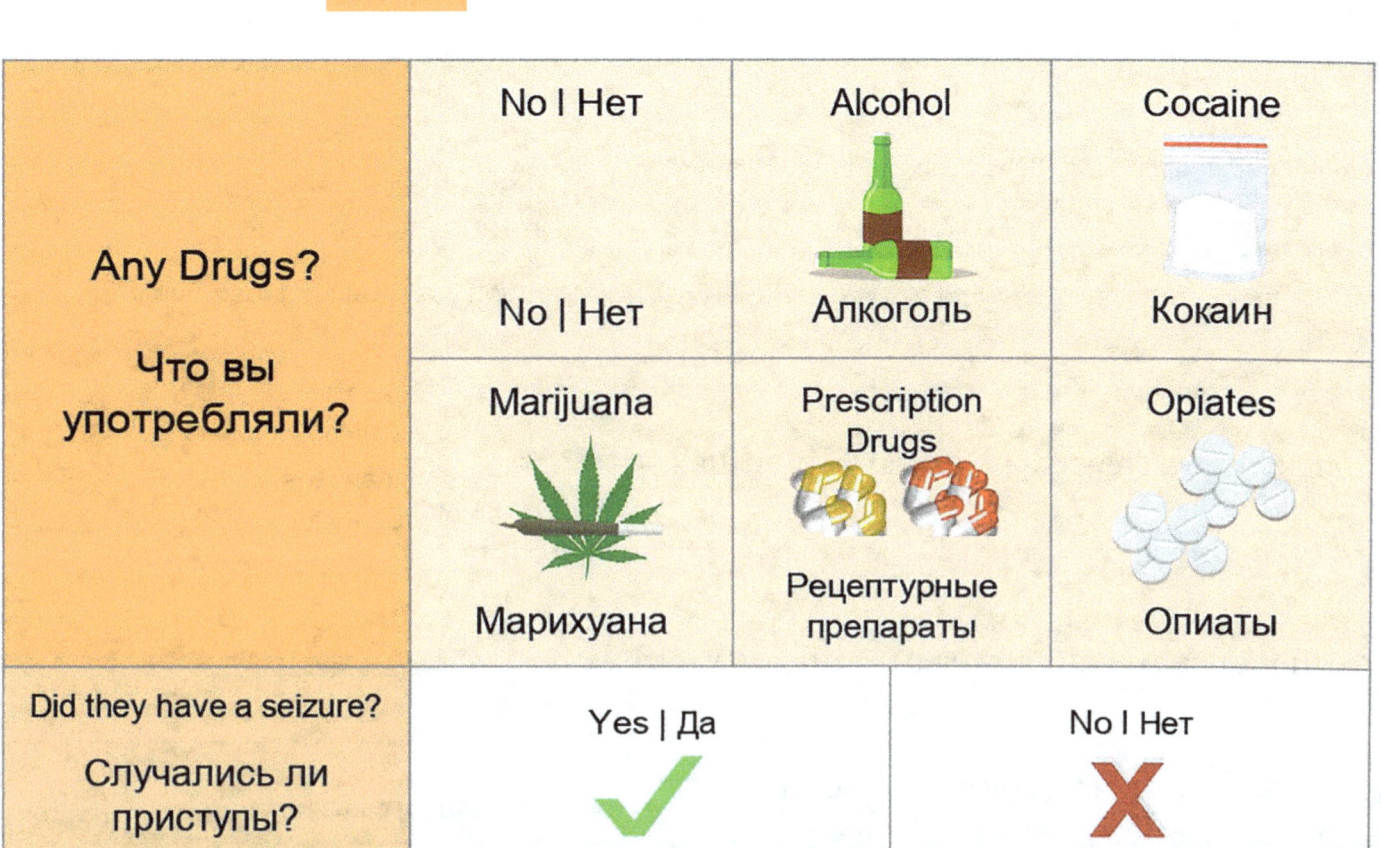

Headache/Dizziness

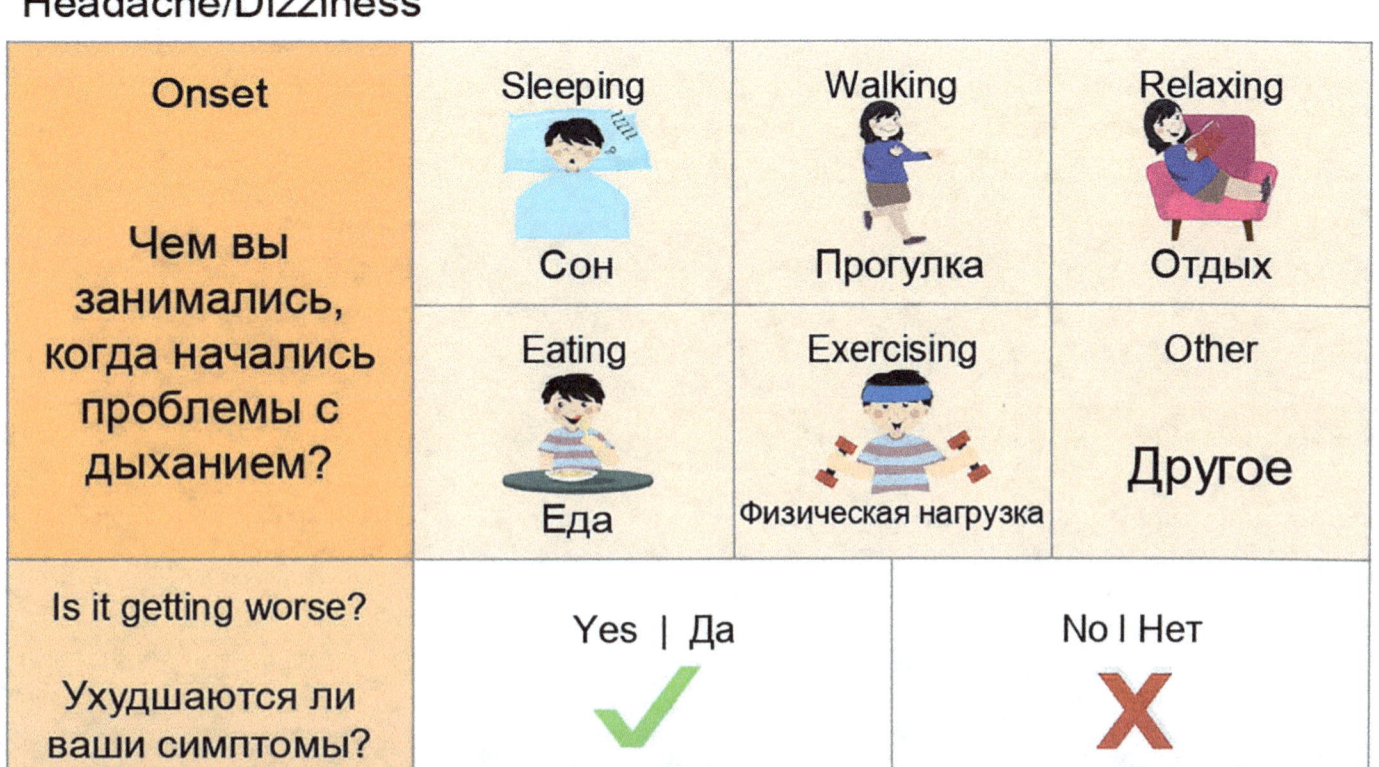

Onset	Sleeping	Walking	Relaxing
	Сон	Прогулка	Отдых
Чем вы занимались, когда начались проблемы с дыханием?	Eating	Exercising	Other
	Еда	Физическая нагрузка	Другое
Is it getting worse?	Yes | Да		No I Нет
Ухудшаются ли ваши симптомы?	✓		X

Time Как давно начали проявляться симптомы?	10 Mins 10 минут	Half Hour Полчаса	1 Hour 1 час
	2 Hours 2 часа	3 Hours 3 часа	>4 Hours Более 4 часов

Has this ever happened before? Случалось ли подобное раньше?	Yes | Да ✔	No | Нет ✗
Do you take your prescribed medications? Принимаете ли вы прописанные лекарства?	Yes | Да ✔	No | Нет ✗

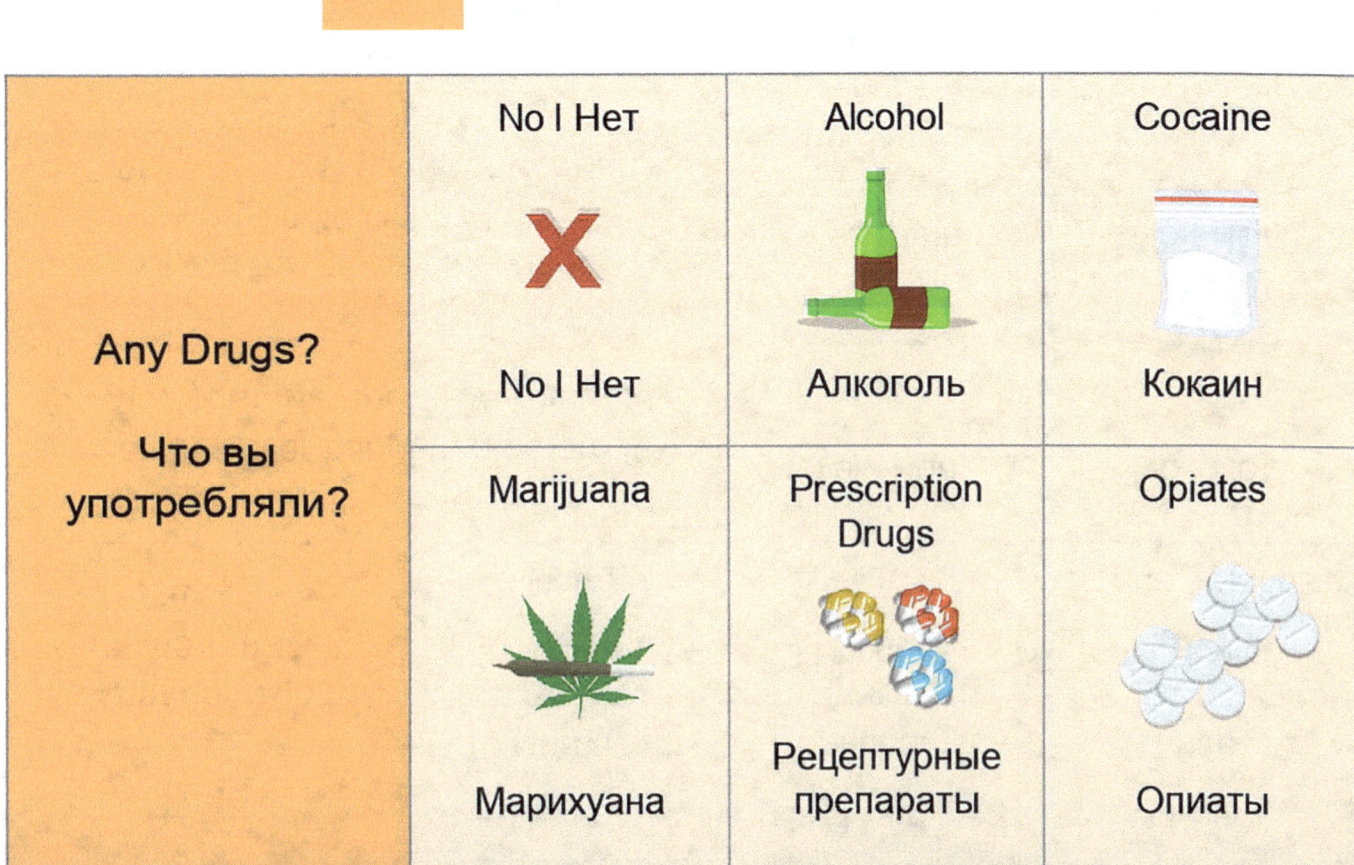

Other complaints? **Беспокоит что-то еще?**	Chest Pain Боль в груди	Abdominal Pain Боль в животе
No I Нет **X**	Shortness of Breath Проблемы с дыханием	Nausea/Vomiting Тошнота и рвота
Other pain **Другие боли**	Syncope Обморок	Headache/Dizziness Головокружение / Головные боли

Fall

Where are you hurting? Где у вас болит?	No Injuries Нет травм		Can you point to where it hurts? Пожалуйста, покажите, что у вас болит	
Time Как давно начали проявляться симптомы?	10 Mins 10 минут	Half Hour Полчаса	1 Hour 1 час	
	2 Hours 2 часа	3 Hours 3 часа	>4 Hours Более 4 часов	
Did you lose consciousness? Вы теряли сознание?	Yes | Да For how long? Как долго вы были без сознания?		No I Нет Are they behaving normal now? Можно ли сказать, что сейчас пациент ведет себя нормально?	

Height of Fall?	1 Feet Полметра	2-3 Feet Полметра-метр	4-5 Feet 1-1,5 метра
Высота падения	6-10 Feet 2-3 метра	11-15 Feet 3-5 метров	>20 Feet >6 метров
Why did you fall?	Trip & Fall/Rolled out of Bed Оступился / Упал с кровати		Weakness/Dizziness Слабость / Головокружение
Почему вы упали?	Fainting/Syncope Обморок		Other Reason Другая причина
Are you on any blood thinning medications? Принимаете ли вы антикоагулянты?	Yes/Да Can we see the medications? Можно взглянуть на эти препараты?		No I Нет. Can we see the medications? Можно ли взглянуть на эти препараты?

Trauma

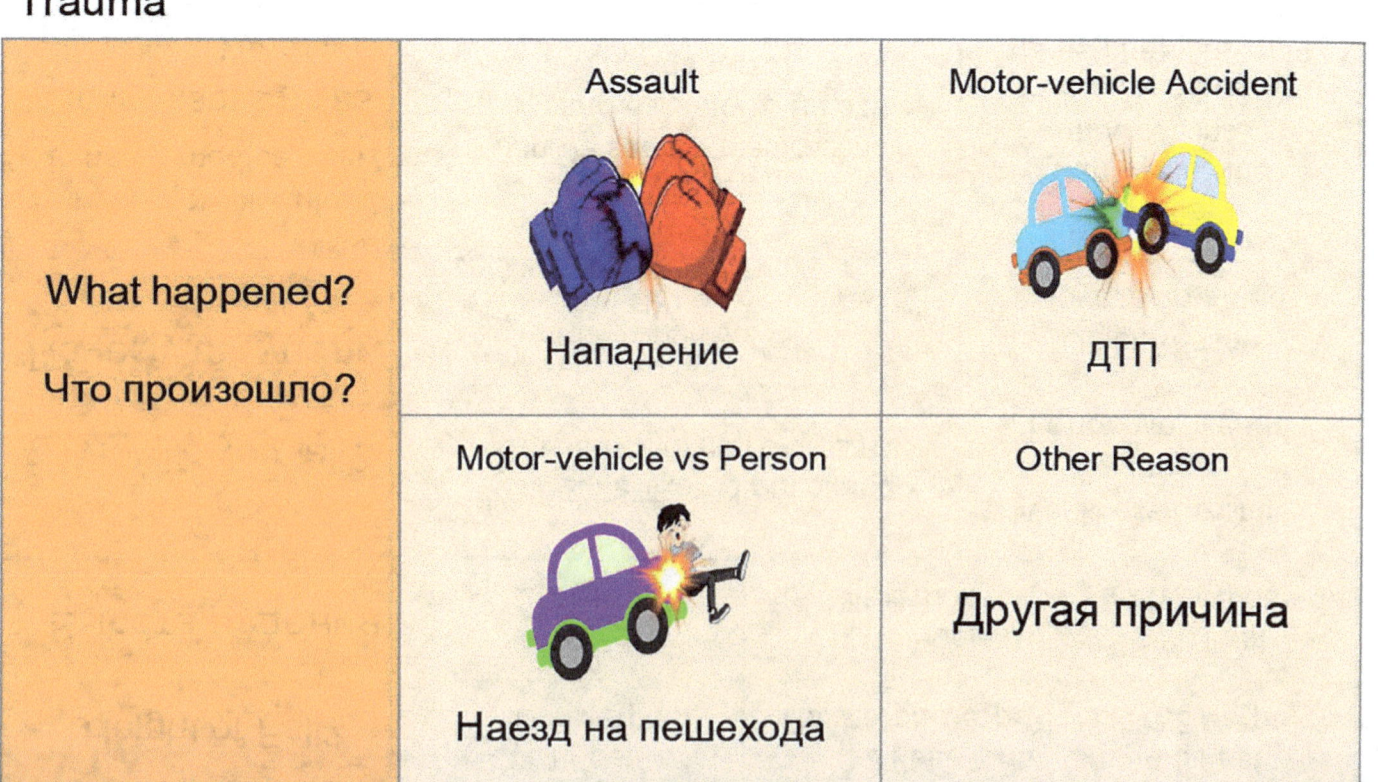

What happened? **Что произошло?**	Assault Нападение	Motor-vehicle Accident ДТП
	Motor-vehicle vs Person Наезд на пешехода	Other Reason Другая причина

Where are you hurting? Где у вас болит?	No Injuries Нет травм		Can you point to where it hurts? Пожалуйста, покажите, что у вас болит	
Time Как давно начали проявляться симптомы?	10 Mins 10 минут	Half Hour Полчаса	1 Hour 1 час	
	2 Hours 2 часа	3 Hours 3 часа	>4 Hours Более 4 часов	
Did you lose consciousness? Вы теряли сознание?	Yes | Да For how long? Как долго вы были без сознания?		No I Нет Are they behaving normal now? Можно ли сказать, что сейчас пациент ведет себя нормально?	

Were you wearing your seatbelt? Вы были пристегнуты?	Yes | Да ✔	No I Нет ✘
Speed of Vehicle С какой скоростью двигалось транспортное средство?	5-10 MPH 5-15 км/ч	10-15 MPH 15-25 км/ч	15-20 MPH 25-30 км/ч
	20-30 MPH 30-50 км/ч	30-40 MPH 50-65 км/ч	Above 50 MPH Более 80 км/ч

Are you on any blood thinning medications? Принимаете ли вы антикоагулянты?	Yes/Да Can we see the medications? Можно ли взглянуть на эти препараты?	No I Нет. Can we see the medications? Можно ли взглянуть на эти препараты?

Miscellaneous Questions

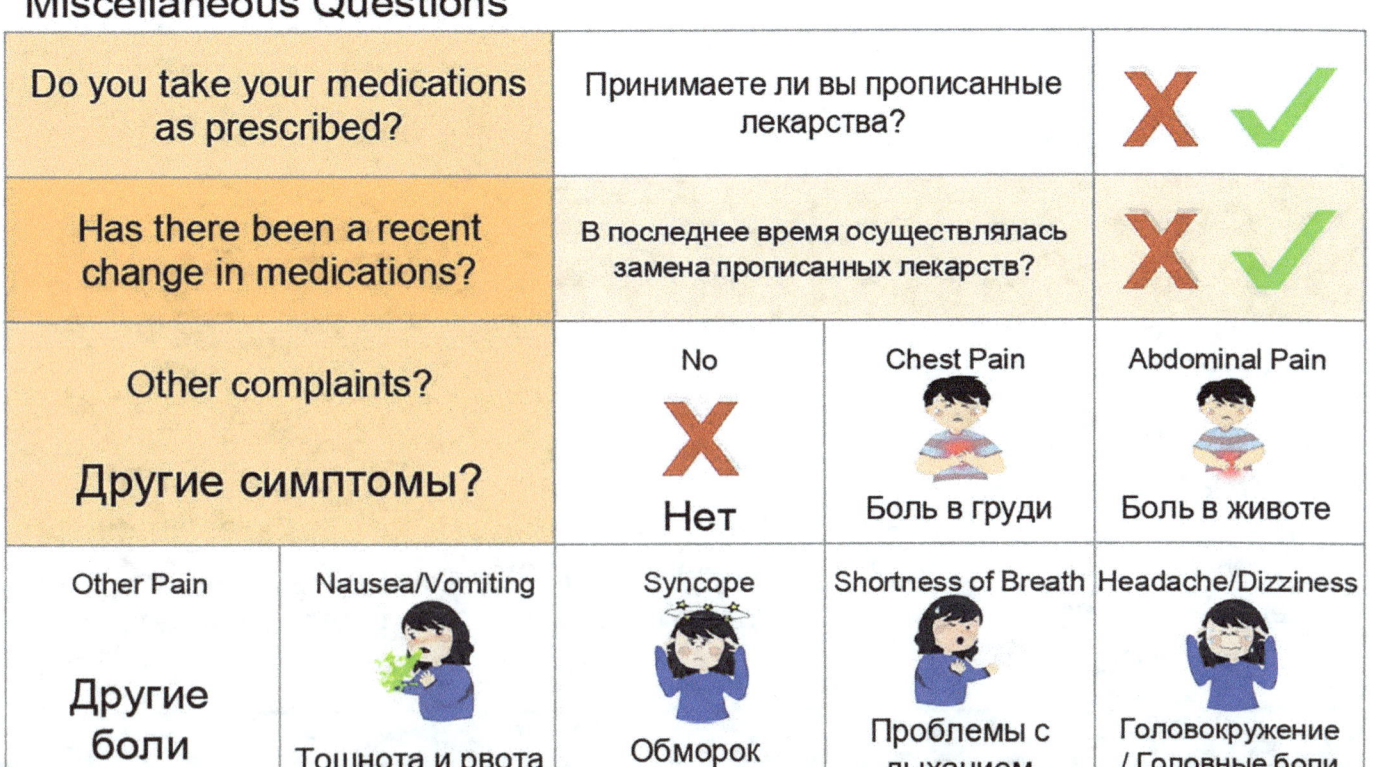

Do you take your medications as prescribed?	Принимаете ли вы прописанные лекарства?	X ✓		
Has there been a recent change in medications?	В последнее время осуществлялась замена прописанных лекарств?	X ✓		
Other complaints? Другие симптомы?	No X Нет	Chest Pain Боль в груди	Abdominal Pain Боль в животе	
Other Pain Другие боли	Nausea/Vomiting Тошнота и рвота	Syncope Обморок	Shortness of Breath Проблемы с дыханием	Headache/Dizziness Головокружение / Головные боли

When was the last time you ate something?	10 Mins 10 минут	Half Hour Полчаса	1 Hour 1 час
Как давно вы ели в последний раз?	2 Hours 2 часа	3 Hours 3 часа	>4 Hours Более 4 часов
Have you ever felt this way before?	Вы когда-нибудь ощущали подобное?	X	✔
Does the patient have a DNR order?	Пациент оформил отказ от реанимации?	X	✔
Do you want to go to the hospital?	Хотите отправиться в больницу?	X	✔

Medical History - История болезни (пожалуйста, выберите)

Asthma	Астма
Atrial Fibrillation	Мерцательная аритмия
Cancer	Рак
COPD	ХОБЛ
Diabetes	Диабет
Hypertension	Гипертония
Heart Failure	Сердечная недостаточность

Liver Problems	Заболевания печени
Myocardial Infarctions	Сердечные приступы в прошлом
Renal Problems	Заболевания почек
Seizures	Припадки
Stroke	Инсульт

Medications - Медикаменты (пожалуйста, выберите)

Aspirin	Аспирин
Atorvastatin	Аторвастатин
Benadryl	Бенадрил
Blood Thinners	Антикоагулянты
Erythromycin	Эритромицин
Fentanyl	Фентанил
Insulin	Инсулин

Ketamine	Кетамин
Metformin	Метформин
Metoprolol	Метопролол
Morphine	Морфин
Penicillin	Пенициллин
Sulfa Drugs	Сульфамидные препараты
Warfarin	Варфарин

Allergies - Аллергии (пожалуйста, выберите)

No Known Drug Allergies	Нет известных мне аллергий
Aspirin	Аспирин
Atorvastatin	Аторвастатин
Benadryl	Бенадрил
Blood Thinners	Антикоагулянты
Erythromycin	Эритромицин
Fentanyl	Фентанил

Ketamine	Кетамин
Metformin	Метформин
Metoprolol	Метопролол
Morphine	Морфин
Penicillin	Пенициллин
Sulfa Drugs	Сульфамидные препараты
Warfarin	Варфарин

Intervention Phrases

I am going to start a IV on you	Я собираюсь поставить вам капельницу
I am going to check your blood sugar	Я собираюсь проверить содержание сахара в крови
I am going to put a collar around your neck	Я собираюсь надеть шейный воротник на вашу шею
I am going to assess your heart, these stickers are going to be on your left chest	Я собираюсь проверить работу вашего сердца. Электроды будут помещены на левую часть вашей груди

I am going to give you a medication. Let me know if your symptoms get better or worst	Я собираюсь дать вам лекарство. Пожалуйста, сообщите, если вам стало лучше/хуже
How are you feeling now? Как вы чувствуете себя в данный момент?	0 2 4 6 8 10